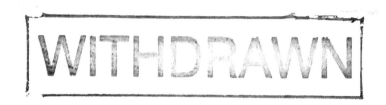

PRACTICE-BASED RESEARCH IN SOCIAL WORK

This unique textbook explores practice-based research (PBR) using numerous practice examples to actively encourage and engage students and practitioners to embrace research as a meaningful support for their practice. While evidence-based practice gives practitioners access to information about "universal" best practices, it does not prioritize practitioner-generated knowledge or promote new research-based interventions relevant to their own practice circumstances as PBR does.

This book discusses the evolution of PBR as a distinct social work research approach, describes its principles and methods and presents a range of exemplars illustrating the application of PBR within different practice methods, and in different practice settings. The chapters cover:

- identifying the research question in a PBR model
- designing a study and identifying a methodology
- sampling
- literature reviews
- gathering data
- ethics
- analyzing data and interpreting results
- putting research into practice.

Viewing the practitioner as central to the research process, and research as a necessary component of practice, this invaluable book emphasizes the seamless integration of practice and research. It is about research *in* social work practice rather than research *on* social work practice. Each chapter includes an overview, an introduction, and a key concepts summary. *Practice-Based Research in Social Work* is a very accessible text suitable for social work students, particularly MSW students, and practitioners.

Sarah-Jane Dodd is an Associate Professor at the Hunter College School of Social Work and the City University of New York Graduate Center, USA. She is also a consulting editor for the *Journal of Teaching in Social Work* and the *Journal of Gay and Lesbian Social Services*.

Irwin Epstein occupies the Helen Rehr Chair in Applied Social Work Research in Health and Mental Health at Hunter College School of Social Work of the City University of New York, USA. He is co-author of several books and numerous articles on social worker professionalization, program evaluation, research utilization and practice-based research. Having introduced this latter concept into the social work literature, his current interest is in exploring clinical data-based research methodology.

To our mothers Pamela Julia Dodd and Rachel Epstein

PRACTICE-BASED RESEARCH IN SOCIAL WORK

A guide for reluctant researchers

Sarah-Jane Dodd and Irwin Epstein

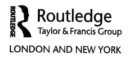

LONDON AND NEW YORK

First published 2012
by Routledge
2 Park Square, Milton Park, Abingdon, Oxon OX14 4RN

Simultaneously published in the USA and Canada
by Routledge
711 Third Avenue, New York, NY 10017

Routledge is an imprint of the Taylor & Francis Group, an informa business

British Library Cataloguing in Publication Data
A catalogue record for this book is available from the British Library

Library of Congress Cataloging in Publication Data
Dodd, Sarah-Jane.
Practice-based research in social work : a guide for reluctant researchers /
Sarah-Jane Dodd and Irwin Epstein.
p. cm.
Includes bibliographical references and index.
1. Social service--Research. 2. Social work education. 3. Social service--
Fieldwork. 4. Social workers--Professional practice. I. Epstein, Irwin. II. Title.
HV11.D633 2012
361.3'2072--dc23   2011022258

ISBN: 978-0-415-56523-3 (hbk)
ISBN: 978-0-415-56524-0 (pbk)
ISBN: 978-0-203-15563-9 (ebk)

Typeset in Sabon
by Bookcraft Limited, Stroud, Gloucestershire

Printed and bound by CPI Group (UK) Ltd, Croydon, CR0 4YY

CONTENTS

LIST OF ILLUSTRATIONS

LIST OF FIGURES

LIST OF BOXES

LIST OF TABLES

ACKNOWLEDGEMENTS

The approach to practice-based research (PBR) taken in this book evolved from a collaborative effort to understand its meaning by research faculty at the Hunter College School of Social Work (HCSSW). Although the research curriculum adopted by the school has been nominally committed to PBR since the early 1980s, over time each instructor developed his or her own interpretation and application of PBR in the classroom. Nonetheless, we all share the same pedagogical philosophy and commitment to research *in* practice rather than *on* practice. Simply stated, we want all students to learn to employ research methods and research ways of thinking in all aspects of their practice.

The suggestion that we write a PBR text originated when Tony Tripodi, former Dean of Ohio State School of Social Work and an eminent research scholar served as the visiting Moses Professor at our school in 2006/07. Bringing together all of Hunter's research faculty, Tony patiently initiated and facilitated meetings, while offering both wise counsel and optimistic encouragement during the early teething stages. We owe a huge "thank you" to Tony for getting us past those cranky yet exciting times.

Based on our early meetings, our research faculty offered a PBR symposium entitled "Meeting the Challenge of Research-Practice Integration: Conducting Practice-Based Research in and with Diverse Communities" at the 2006 Society for Social Work Research (SSWR) conference in San Antonio. Though the seminar was slotted into the last session of the last day of the conference when most conference participants had already left or were heading to the airport and remembering the Alamo, we were pleasantly surprised that so many actually showed and stayed through our two-hour, Sunday morning seminar. Clearly, some research academics were intrigued by our unique orientation to teaching and conducting research.

Colleagues who presented in that PBR seminar and/or were part of those early meetings included Irene Chung, Nancy Feldman, Harriet Goodman, George Patterson, Andrea Savage, Mike Smith and Darrell Wheeler. To them, we owe our gratitiude. As the scope of the project took shape and it became clear that a unified voice was needed most went their separate ways, sinking their teeth into other projects. Still, those early meetings and that seminar helped the two of us to solidify our conceptual thinking. These same colleagues provided ongoing support and encouragement to us as we took the book on as our own.

Reading a co-authored book is a lot easier than writing one. Co-authors have different priorities, life circumstances, career contingencies as well as different styles of writing and working. Dean Jacqueline Mondros at HCSSW granted S.J. a sabbatical in order to move us past the conceptual and into the writing phase of the project. For that S.J. thanks her. A veteran of many sabbaticals and the occupant of the Helen Rehr Chair in Applied Social Work Research at Hunter, I.E. thanks Dean Mondros and Helen Rehr for graciously letting him do what he does whether on or off sabbatical.

Jim Agoli our universally adored computer and IT guy provided invaluable help in transferring research concepts into diagrammatic form. Our editor Grace McInnes lived up to her pledge in allowing us the space and time to hash out conceptual and authorial concerns above adherence to the unrealistic deadlines we ourselves had set. Plus she has a sense of humor. Her assistant James Watson provided clear, efficient and welcome support as we moved through the final stages of the process. We are also grateful that our production editor, Richenda Milton-Daws, was simultaneously thorough, respectful and gentle with our work.

On a personal note S.J. would like to thank Bruce Jansson, Margaret W. Driscoll/ Louise M. Clevenger Professor of Social Policy and Administration at the University of Southern California, an incredible scholar and generous mentor; Professors John Brekke, Bill Meezan and Bob Nishimoto who ignited my love of research during my PhD at the University of Southern California. Gary Mallon, the Julia Lathrop Professor of Child Welfare at HCSSW, a thoughtful, generous and always encouraging colleague and friend; Maddy Petrow-Cohen who exemplified friendship and provided invaluable support throughout; my loving family in England, especially my Mum and Dad who were crazy enough to support my moving to the US in the first place, and who have given unwavering love and support ever since. And my family here in the US, Laura my amazing partner and our two beautiful children Emma and Jack who were always ready to give me support and encouragement or to make me laugh just when I needed it most. Our family brings joy and meaning to my every day.

On an equally personal note, I.E. wishes to thank his loving family, Fran, Becs, Carole, Dan, Molly and Stephen and his buddies Ted Benjamin, George Downs, Jeffrey Harper, Dana Holman, Richard Joelson, Tony Tripodi and George Ziskind for the occasional drinks and loyal friendship during the good and not so good times during which this book was written.

Though she lived to see her 100th birthday this year, this is the first book that Rachel Epstein will not have lived to see published and proudly added to her unread pile of "Irwin's books" just under the TV set. She was his greatest booster though some academic antagonists might say precisely *because* she never read them. "Pay no mind to them" she'd say, "they wish they could write that book."

Of course, our greatest debt is to the countless and initially research "reluctant" social work students and practitioners who trusted us enough to let us join with them as they explored their practice questions in increasingly systematic and thoughtful ways. Their practice-relevant studies exemplify PBR, some of which we discuss throughout this book. Thank you.

Sarah-Jane Dodd and Irwin Epstein

Part 1

Introduction to PBR in social work practice

INTRODUCTION

THIS BOOK'S PURPOSE

For most students, and regretfully the majority of social work practitioners, the words "research" and "practice" occupy opposite ends of a continuum. Indeed, in most students' and practitioners' minds, the terms are generally separated by "versus" – as though they were at opposing corners of the boxing ring.

Nonetheless, the Code of Ethics adopted by the National Association of Social Workers (NASW) in 2008 requires that "Social workers should monitor and evaluate policies, the implementation of programs, and practice interventions" and should promote and facilitate evaluation and research to contribute to the development of knowledge" (p.25). As a result, every NASW member is obliged to incorporate research into her or his practice and ideally to contribute to the development of social work's knowledge base. Whether they do or not is another story.

In reality, compliance with this ethical obligation is left up to the practitioner. And while some social work research professors have argued that those who do not are guilty of "malpractice" (Myers and Thyer, 1997), those of us who teach research but are mindful of realistic constraints recognize that threats and punishments are no ways to win the hearts and minds of our research students as future practitioners. We do, however, think it is vital for social workers, and in particular for social work practitioners to be engaged in research, so that questions can be generated from a social work perspective and explored in social work settings. If social workers do not engage in research then we have to rely on other professions to generate knowledge for us, something that we have relied on for a long time. So our insistence on the importance of practitioners being involved in research is so that our research questions stay relevant and realistic and add a social work practice perspective to knowledge-building.

Consistent with the position taken by NASW is the recently adopted Educational Policy and Accreditation Standards 2.1.6 of the Council on Social Work Education (CSWE). CSWE, which accredits all Baccalaureate and Master's degree programs in social work, requires that all social work students be prepared to "engage in research-informed practice and practice-informed research" (CSWE, 2008, p.5). So whether you want to or not, as a social work student you are obliged to take at least one course in research.

Though the foregoing requirements are relatively new, the aversion of social work students to research is an old story. Despite our capacity to use research comfortably in other areas of our lives (such as when choosing a graduate school, or buying a computer) social workers balk at the idea of one or more research classes. Whether fuelled by a fear of statistics (Wilson and Rosenthal, 1993), ethical opposition to research requirements, an objection to reducing individual clients to computer categories, resistance to overly broad cultural stereotypes, the perception of research irrelevance or the simple preference to be studying something else, it is safe to say that most social work students are "reluctant" to enroll in a required research course.

Indeed, over a decade ago, Epstein (1987) characterized social work students as "research reluctants". Writing about the social work research requirement, he noted:

> No other part of the social work curriculum has been so consistently received by students with as much groaning, moaning, eye-rolling, bad-mouthing, hyperventilation and waiver-strategizing as the research courses.
>
> (Epstein, 1987, p.71)

That was true then and, as Harder (2010) suggests, it is true today. Hence, those of us who teach research are united in a commitment to integrate practice and research. We differ however in how we try to do that. Some emphasize the ethical obligation to use the most current results of "gold standard" social work research studies so that clients receive interventions that are shown by these studies to be most effective (Gambrill, 2006). These social work researchers are identified with the evidence-based practice (EBP) movement in social work (Kirk and Reid, 2002).

The influence of this movement has extended well beyond the classroom to many social work agencies wherein "manualized" interventions based on prior research are incorporated into how social workers are expected to practice. Although there is debate among academics about how much freedom this gives or should give practitioners to be creative in their practice, manualization of practice has not been welcomed by many practitioners. While they would not disagree with its intent – to better serve clients – they object to the way it encroaches on their professional autonomy and overrides practice instincts (Epstein, 2011).

Elsewhere, Epstein (2009) has been critical of EBP for treating practitioners solely as research consumers rather than as practitioner-researchers and as potential contributors to research knowledge for the profession. Similar to the approach taken by Harder (2010) in teaching MSW research courses, he has written about the ways practitioners and PhD students in social work can "mine" routinely available agency data to inform their practice decision-making as well as to contribute to the knowledge base of social work.

The purpose of this book is to broaden that perspective and demonstrate the many ways in which research concepts and simple and ethically-acceptable research projects can contribute to the quality of your practice as a social work student and as a future professional. In other words, our purpose is to make research more "practice-friendly", help you see it as such and, in so doing to reduce your reluctance to use it. There, we've said it!

At the same time, it should be clear that our intention is not to make research so appealing that you abandon practice altogether and decide to become a research professor like us – unless of course you want to. We've happily spent our careers doing just that and loving it. But in this book, our joint mission is to keep the word "practitioner" first and foremost in every research discussion. For you as well as for us, that rightfully means always keeping your clients' best interests as well as your primary aspiration to be a social worker rather than a researcher firmly in mind.

Given students' research reluctance mentioned earlier, achieving this purpose is a tall order. There are lots of required research texts on the shelves of libraries and school bookstores. Almost as many are in bookstores' remainder bins, on student bulletin-boards and on eBay for resale until a new edition gets assigned. We're hoping that this one is a "keeper".

More significantly, we're hoping that the concepts and techniques discussed and described in this book will become integrated into your practice as a student, as a future social work practitioner and throughout your career. Many of the concepts and techniques have been around as long as we have. What's new, however, is how they are put into practice. That is the essence of practice-based research (PBR).

WHAT IS PBR?

Simply stated, PBR is research conducted by practitioners for practice purposes. The goal is to inform practice and practitioners throughout the research process. Thus, PBR emphasizes immediate practical applications by practitioner-researchers who conduct PBR studies. These studies may be conducted by individual social workers, teams of social workers or multi-disciplinary teams, with or without research consultation. When that consultation is available however, it is fully collaborative rather than dominated by research considerations (see Chapter 13, Figure 13.7). As a result, it maintains its focus on the decision-making requirements, the agency context and existing policies within which the social worker must practice – in other words, the practice reality. In addition, PBR takes into account the ethical priorities of the practitioner who initiates the study.

This sounds complex and it is. In that regard it requires that you, the practitioner-researcher, possess a flexible repertoire of research techniques and a wide-ranging research vocabulary. On the other hand, it is quite simple because PBR is so pragmatic. Just like the time-honoured social work practice principle of starting where the client is, PBR starts where the worker is and asks how research can help take the individual client, the group, the program or the community to the next step. Sometimes this may require some additional research consultation, often not.

We're not talking "rocket science" here. Nor are we talking running lab rats through mazes. We're talking about relatively simple modes of systematic inquiry that will inform and improve your work and your understanding of your work. But while the research itself is relatively simple, the reality in which it is conducted and to which it is applied is complex. Just like the social work reality in which you have your field placement and like any practice setting in which you will work post-graduation, the context for PBR is complex and dynamic.

A more detailed definition of PBR and a more complex model of practitioner-researcher collaboration will be presented later in the book. At this point what is most important for you to understand is that the findings of practitioner-initiated PBR are intended primarily for use in a specific practice and agency context. They may be studies to plan a new program, to better understand and/or evaluate an existing program, or all three. Or they may focus on a single client, a family or a group. The problems or phenomena that these studies address emerge directly from practice and provide "evidence-informed" answers to practitioners' questions. Consequently, PBR is never about research for its own sake. Hence if you think of practice and research on a continuum rather than as a dichotomy (and that would be good), PBR comes closer to the practice end of that continuum.

Still, once PBR studies are completed, their methods and findings might have application and be of interest to practitioners and researchers elsewhere. That's why some PBR studies begin with a purely local intention and are subsequently published or presented at conferences. All the better when that happens. But they never begin with the question "Wouldn't it be interesting to know?" Instead, they require a practice-based reason *why* it would be interesting to know from a practice perspective, and *how* that information will be used in practice. So, PBR is all about applied rather than basic research. And as a practitioner-researcher (which is how we hope you will view yourself at the end of this book) the application of your PBR studies will be directly to your social work practice.

THE PRACTITIONER-RESEARCHER OR THE RESEARCHER-PRACTITIONER?

In our unending pursuit of just the right way to integrate science and social work practice, academics have championed several practice–research integration "movements" (Kirk and Reid, 2002; Tripodi and Lalayants, 2008). Their remains litter the roadside of social work research.

Most prominent today is the evidence-based practice (EBP) movement. Simply stated, EBP is about giving priority to those interventions that have been shown to be effective through the "best possible evidence", understood by proponents of EBP as, randomized controlled experiments. While some EBP opponents argue that many significant social work interventions for practical and ethical reasons do not lend themselves to experimental studies (e.g., provision of necessary material services, complex psycho-dynamic interventions, etc.), EBP is currently in its ascendancy in many schools of social work as well as many social agencies. In fact, in many practice contexts, governmental funding is currently also linked to an EBP philosophy.

Still, the roots of EBP in social work run deep and can be traced back to the mid-1970s when Briar (1979) championed the concept of the "scientist-practitioner". Very much like EBP today, the scientist-practitioner as Briar saw it was one who:

- Identified client problems in measurable ways;
- Chose interventions after systematically reviewing the research literature;
- Gave preference to single interventions that were shown to be most effective through research; and then
- Evaluated their effectiveness using a "single-system" design approach.

The latter did not involve classical experimentation but stuck very close to the logic of experimentation. In other words, while all clients received interventions and none were randomly assigned to control groups and denied services, practitioners were encouraged, first to conduct "baseline measures" of client needs over several sessions before intervening to establish that these were real and not diminishing on their own; and second, to periodically "withdraw" interventions and then re-introduce them in order to establish their measurable effectiveness. Clearly, this approach gave priority to the role of "scientist" rather than to other more service-oriented conceptions of social work.

At the time, many students, practitioners and social agencies rejected this model of practice–research integration. Not surprisingly, it conjured up objectionable images of passionless social workers in lab coats treating clients as experimental objects rather than as human beings with complex problems that required complex interventions.

Today, some EBP proponents still advocate practitioner use of single-system designs to evaluate the effectiveness of individual and program interventions (McCracken and Marsh, 2008). They also emphasize the importance of the systematic review of the research literature by the practitioner or by someone who does it for the practitioner. More generally, however, EBP advocates simply assume that those interventions that demonstrate "evidence-based" effectiveness will be effective wherever, whenever and with whomever they are applied. So, while they do not use the term "scientist-practitioner" *per se*, they clearly give priority to the practitioner's reliance on scientific research in choosing interventions. In fact, they assert that anything else places clients at grave risk.

Our PBR approach is quite different. We do not deny the importance of critically consulting the research literature. In fact, we strongly encourage students and practitioners to consult and critically assess the research literature whenever they confront an individual, group or community problem. However, we emphasize the primacy and complexity of the practitioner's role – much of which extends beyond narrowly assessing, intervening and evaluating client problems. Instead, this book treats research as simply a tool to inform and support practitioner decision-making and client service provision. Hence it is no accident that in our model of practice–research integration the word "practitioner" comes before the word "researcher". As a result, throughout the book we will be suggesting how a PBR approach to research differs from a research-based practice (RBP) approach.

THE "ART" OF STRATEGIC COMPROMISE

Social work is as much an art as it is a science. Although many in the EBP movement would prefer that it be entirely the latter, most practitioners emphasize the former. Similarly, the task of integrating practice and research is as much an art as a science. Those who emphasize the science talk about "translational research" and how to find ways to incorporate the findings of science into practice in such a way as to preserve the integrity of the science (Brekke, Ell and Palinkas, 2007). In that debate, we take a "softer" position, firmly believing that social work can and should never be entirely a science. Human beings, social arrangements and different cultures are just too complex to be reduced to a set of scientific principles, research findings and practice interventions. So, throughout this book, we emphasize the importance of "strategic compromise" in making use of research concepts, techniques and findings in integrating research into your practice.

In our "practice" as research teachers and research consultants, we have found strategic compromise to be essential to our success. It makes it possible to take the best of science but to apply it in a practical and realistic manner, understanding and accepting its limitations as well as the ways it improves our prior understanding. Ironically, even the most ardent, "gold standard" researchers routinely compromise their research ideal in order to get their studies done. This may involve oversimplifying the problems they study, choosing sample populations that are not ideal, continuing their studies to completion despite significant subject drop-out, etc. Hopefully, they acknowledge these issues when discussing their "study limitations".

Instead, just as practitioners must adjust their practice ideals to the reality of the client's situation, the agency context in which they are working and the social policies that constrain or support their interventions, we consider strategic compromise as an essential tool in improving practice through research. In conducting PBR, it is elevated to a basic principle rather than disguised or minimized. As a result, strategic compromise is a theme that runs through this entire book.

STRUCTURE OF THE BOOK

For obvious reasons, this book begins with a chapter on the evolution and underlying principles of PBR. If nothing else, we try to be logical and systematic – after all, we are researchers. But we may try to slip in a joke or two now and then as well. We're human beings and we want this to be fun for you as well as for us. We're also realistic. Several decades of combined teaching of research has taught us that, in teaching research, sometimes the best student feedback we can expect in our course evaluations is the oft-repeated sentiment "I thought this course would be agony, but you made the subject tolerable." After reading this book, we're hoping for evaluations that contain the words "interesting", "fun" and, most important, "useful".

Following the brief introductory chapter about PBR, the book gives most of its attention to the PBR process – how to get started, how to do it, how to use it. In so doing, the book admittedly covers topics covered in most other social work research texts, such as research designs, sampling, research ethics, etc. Booooooring perhaps? We hope not.

What's different about our book is how these topics are discussed and when they are discussed. So, for example, many research texts and many research teachers begin with locating and reviewing existing research literature. Similarly, EBP assumes that that's where the practitioner begins. But as experienced PBR researchers and research-consultants, we know that that's not where studies begin. Instead, they begin with a practice problem and some serious thinking about how some systematic data gathering (doesn't have to be quantitative, but could be), analysis (doesn't have to use the computer, but might), interpretation (doesn't have to rely on some elaborate theory, or prior research studies, unless of course they help) and utilization (often the most challenging, but that's why you're doing this to begin with) might be beneficial to practice and program decision-making.

What we've just described is the entire process of PBR in particular and applied research in general. So, it's no accident that it's not until Chapter 5, that we discuss the literature review process. Returning to the beginnings of the PBR process, however, Chapter 2 is about how to identify a practice problem for which some PBR might come in handy. Chapter 3 discusses the different purposes of PBR studies, while Chapter 4, on PBR designs, looks at how you might structure a PBR study in such a way as it "honors practice protocols". By the latter phrase we mean, doesn't intrude on your practice and/or conflict with your clients' needs. (Remember, this isn't about doing research just to do research.)

As we indicated above, Chapter 5 focuses on review of available research literature. Not unlike student course evaluations, some PBR studies (e.g., patient satisfaction surveys) may be conducted and meaningfully used without the benefit of a literature review. But why go through the hassle of developing an original questionnaire when someone has already done it for you? How do your findings compare with findings for similar patients in other programs? How do others translate their findings into practice and program implications? If you are interested in these and other questions, then a literature review can come in handy as well.

Chapter 6 is about what kind of data-gathering methodology (*aka* method) you will use. Will it be quantitative, qualitative or mixed methodology (*aka* both)? Ideally, upon finishing this book and the research course for which you are likely to be reading it, you will feel equally comfortable with all three options and use them as the PBR problem requires. Deciding about which also takes into account the costs as well as the benefits of each, and good PBR involves thinking about how to minimize the costs (e.g., time, money, intrusiveness, etc.) as well as maximizing data quality and comprehensiveness. Here, as in every aspect of PBR decision-making, "strategic compromise" comes into play.

Chapters 7 and 8 discuss ways of gathering qualitative and quantitative data respectively. The emphasis for both chapters is about maximizing the quality of the data you gather without disrupting or violating your practice commitments. Here again, the concepts are basic to every form of research and are not new. What's different is how "strategic compromise" plays a role in making decisions about maximizing quality and minimizing costs.

Chapter 9 is about sampling concepts and techniques, which are useful in every study (qualitative, quantitative or mixed) when resource requirements and other practical considerations prevent you from studying the entire population that you are interested in knowing something practice-relevant about. Although sampling concepts and techniques have changed very little over the years, they are incredibly useful and practical. That's why they haven't changed. Computer programs can make certain aspects of sampling easier, but the basic concepts remain the same.

One place in which "compromise" of any kind does not have a proper place in PBR is ethics. Chapter 10 is about research ethics and the protection of human subjects. Schools of social work and just about every social agency have a committee or organizational process to protect individuals who are subjects in research studies. Sometimes these are referred to as Institutional Review Boards (IRBs) or Ethics Committees or Human Subjects Committees. Whatever their label, and however cumbersome their process, their purpose is very important. This is particularly important in social work research studies, which may be about highly sensitive information that potentially makes our clients extremely vulnerable. PBR is flexible about other things, but it takes ethics very seriously. However, as discussed in Chapter 6, there are ethical ways of conducting research on highly sensitive topics that do not place respondents in jeopardy or place an undue burden on them.

Chapters 11 and 12 are about data analysis that you can do entirely on your own or with a research consultant. Chapter 11 focuses on strategies for analyzing qualitative data, and Chapter 12 focuses on analyzing quantitative data. Both chapters are written with the full intent that any social work practitioner (even you) can develop the skills necessary to analyze PBR data. This is because, even if you do decide that you would like some outside help, it's important for you to know how and why you want further consultation so that you remain in charge of your study, your data and its purposes.

Finally, Chapter 13 is about interpreting your findings and disseminating them, that is to say putting them into practice and communicating them to others. Sharing your findings with others is a crucial part of the PBR purpose of research that informs practice. These "significant" others or what researchers refer to as "stakeholders" may be other professionals in your own agency or those in other agencies or the profession at large. Chapter 13 also discusses using research consultants in a collaborative manner. Once you have mastered the basic components of the PBR process, you will be able to approach research consultation in a truly collaborative way keeping your research consultants accountable to you and your research purpose. Ultimately then, this book is about empowering practitioners to conduct and learn from research and to contribute to knowledge rather than to feel intimidated by research and/or researchers. Our objective is to help you become more than an educated consumer, but rather a producer of knowledge about social work practice as well. A tall order perhaps, but years of successfully teaching PBR has convinced us both that you are up to it.

Chapter 1

Evolution and definition of PBR

Purpose

This chapter offers a comprehensive definition of practice-based research (PBR) and describes how and why PBR came about. It goes on to distinguish PBR from evidence-based practice (EBP) but in so doing, emphasizes the mutually-reinforcing contribution of both. Both have strengths as well as limitations, and while this book unapologetically advocates a PBR approach, in this chapter we acknowledge PBR's limitations as well as its strengths. In conclusion however, we argue that PBR is a much better match to the values and normative commitments of social work practitioners and students like you than — other forms of practice-research integration. Finally, we suggest that this is also true for the clients and communities that you serve.

INTRODUCTION

In the introductory chapter, we loosely defined PBR as research conducted by practitioners for practice purposes. Elsewhere, Epstein (2001, p.17) defined it more precisely as:

> the use of research-inspired principles, designs and information gathering techniques within existing forms of practice to answer questions that emerge from practice in ways that inform practice.

That's a mouthful, but it contains within it all the elements that make PBR different from other forms of research and makes explicit how this book differs from other research texts.

Working backwards (and this is often the case with PBR), it should be clear that its ultimate purpose is to inform practice. In other words, PBR is applied research rather than basic research – that is, its primary emphasis is on utilization rather than knowledge for its own sake. As a result, it is a kind of research that is conducted close to practice even if its contributions are relatively modest. Something as simple as systematically finding out about the food, program or entertainment preferences of a senior client group may not constitute a major contribution to knowledge more generally, but it may make the difference between group attendance and total washout. Of course, your goals for the group may go far beyond providing food or entertainment, but as a group worker you can't achieve those more lofty goals if no one attends your group.

Continuing in reverse gear is the reference to "questions that emerge from practice". In research language, Epstein is describing an inductive rather than a deductive approach to generating the questions that drive the research. In other words, rather than beginning with very abstract theoretical notions or hypotheses that are tested through research, PBR attempts to answer questions that come directly from practice decision-making requirements facing the social worker – for example, who am I serving and what are their needs? Am I providing the services I am committed to providing? How effective are those services in the eyes of my clients and how satisfied are they with them? Should I continue doing what I've been doing, or should I change?

Perhaps the most important distinguishing element in our definition is "within existing forms of practice". While PBR emphasizes inventiveness and flexibility (some might say it is too flexible and not scientifically "rigorous" enough), the one unyielding principle in PBR is that you never compromise established practice principles in order to conduct research. So, finding ways to conduct research within existing agency rules, client preferences, and practice wisdom is perhaps the ultimate challenge of PBR. The central question that PBR poses for the practitioner is "How can I be more systematic in my approach to using information on behalf of my clients without compromising their wishes or my ethical and value commitments?"

The remaining portion of the definition refers to "the use of research-inspired principles, designs and information gathering techniques" and the rest of this book will tell you what those principles, designs and information-gathering techniques are. Our hope is that you will not only learn what they are, but incorporate them into your PBR "repertoire" so that you can mix and match them as the practice situation requires. It might require a self-administered quantitative questionnaire in one situation or a qualitative focus group in another. It might involve combining available statistical information with individual interviews in another.

Once you are confident in your mastery of these research techniques and you are comfortably grounded in your value commitments, you can use these techniques to reflect upon, evaluate and possibly change your practice, or even that of your agency. Whichever you do, it will now be based more on "practice-based evidence" than on "practitioner intuition" or going entirely "with your gut".

HOW PBR CAME ABOUT

Those of you who sail will know that the term "coming about" refers to the moment when whoever is captaining the ship signals that the boat is changing its tack, when the sail is repositioned and everyone in the way of the changing sail must duck in order to avoid a powerful hit on the head. Perhaps it is an apt metaphor because while the PBR "tack" is different from other approaches to practice–research integration, all of us are trying to get to the same place – that is the provision of better service to our clients and our client communities. But PBR takes a slightly different route from most academic researchers and conventional textbooks. Since you are probably reading this book because your research professor assigned it, we're assuming you won't get smacked on the head for doing so.

To sail a bit further on our new tack, PBR "came about" as a reaction to conventional ways of thinking about, writing about and teaching social work research. After years of hearing academic colleagues complain about and reading lots of papers documenting workers' and social work students' dislike of research, Epstein (1995) began thinking seriously about why they disliked it, and looking for alternative routes to the same place that everyone else wanted to go to. Rather than "blaming the students" (who often thought of themselves as "the victim"), he wondered whether there was a better way to teach research, and to engage practicing social workers in research. Somehow, the continuing stream of criticism reminded him of the *My Fair Lady* song in which Professor Henry Higgins, who is trying to teach his cockney protégée Eliza Doolittle to speak "proper" English, famously laments "Why can't a woman be more like a man?"

Charmed by the tongue-in-cheek message of that song, but struck by its parallel in social work research education, Epstein (1996) published an article which he ironically subtitled "Or, Why can't a social worker be more like a researcher?" In this and subsequent writings, he began trying to understand the legitimate reasons why social workers resist approaches to practice that are dominated by research considerations. There are many.

Not surprisingly, his article drew some criticism from advocates of research-based approaches to practice, including one who noted that in his very choice of music, Epstein was revealing how anachronistic and "behind the times" his views were (Ivanoff *et al.*, 1997). However, not everyone thought that PBR was passé, especially not practitioners. In fact, many felt it was a welcome change and a more collaborative approach to knowledge generation. Students especially responded favorably.

So, based on the positive response by practitioners and students to his work, Epstein continued to chart his PBR course alone (Epstein, 2001, 2005, 2007, 2009, 2010) and in collaboration with a few like-minded academics and practitioners (Grasso and Epstein, 1992; Epstein and Blumenfield, 2001; Peake *et al.*, 2005; Vonk, Tripodi and Epstein, 2006). Along the way, we coordinated with our research colleagues at Hunter to put on a symposium at the Society for Social Work Research (SSWR) annual conference, entitled "Meeting the Challenge of Research-Practice Integration: Conducting Practice-Based Research in and with Diverse Communities" (Dodd and Epstein, 2006). The positive but cautious response from colleagues suggested that there was indeed room for PBR in the social work research ocean, especially in the classroom. And so, discovering that they were employing similar approaches to teaching research and in research consultation with social work agencies (Dobrof *et al.*, 2006; Dodd and Meezan, 2009), Dodd and Epstein decided to set out together writing this book.

Although those first PBR articles and those on "research reluctance" were published decades ago, academics are still complaining about social workers' weak research profile and social work students' resistance to research. Hence, in a recent issue of *Research on Social Work Practice*, arguably the most prominent and dominant research journal in the field, Stoesz (2010) bemoans an academic career marred by frustration and spent dealing with students' math anxiety and practitioners' rejection of rigorous research.

Incorporating his personal lament into a review of a new EBP book, Stoesz (2010) calls for a major "paradigm shift" in social work from "pre-scientific activity" (presumably what social workers now do) to EBP. Like other research academics who have been critical of social work practitioners, Stoesz (2010, pp.329–30) comments:

> EBP represents a challenge to social work as a prescientific activity, a muddle of humanism, psychoanalysis, and most recently postmodernism. For proponents of EBP, little of social work, as it has evolved, makes much logical sense; its validity is based ultimately on the "authority" of practitioners as opposed to any independent rational assessment of efficacy. In the absence of evidence, social work is a grab bag of good intentions … just as likely to inflict harm as benefit.

Never once, does Stoesz question whether the scientific movement might be doing something wrong, or be taking the wrong tack. Maybe *My Fair Lady* isn't so out of date after all?

Unfortunately, this theme of criticizing practitioners with much less charm runs through much of the prevailing rhetoric of EBP (Epstein, 2011). It is built on the very extreme assumption that anything that social workers do that isn't based on rigorously researched quantitative findings and the accumulation of the products of randomized controlled experiments is dangerous and potentially harmful.

This position is expressed in extremis by Eileen Gambrill, one of the most prolific EBP advocates, who in an invited article in the same journal issue as Stoesz's book review, argues that all criticisms of EBP are mere "propaganda ploys" to support the "quackery, fraud and corruption" that in her eyes characterize conventional social work practice today (Gambrill, 2010). To her, criticism of EBP constitutes "censorship" by people who "have no concern for truth, only to create credibility" through "guile and charm" (p.304).

In writing this book, our intention is not to take an equally extreme position opposing EBP but rather to assert an appreciative understanding and respect for what practitioners do. We simply employ logic and good sense, and our familiarity with research principles and techniques to present a more "practice-friendly" alternative that can live side-by-side with EBP. Rather than continue in this seemingly futile "we versus them" approach to research and practice, our intention is to offer a more collaborative and mutually appreciative approach whereby social work students and practitioners can become independent producers of social work knowledge and whereby practitioners working together with academic researchers can become co-creators of social work knowledge. But before we do, let's first explore some of the major underlying differences between PBR and EBP.

DISTINGUISHING PBR AND EBP

In 2001 Epstein contrasted PBR with what he referred to generally as "research-based practice" (RBP). EBP is only one model of RBP, but it is the one currently in academic ascendancy. In that article, Epstein (2001, p.17) defined RBP (as opposed to PBR) as:

> The use of research-based concepts, theories, designs and data-gathering instruments to structure practice so that hypotheses concerning cause-effect relationships between social work interventions and outcomes may be rigorously tested.

That definition was conceived based upon Briar's model of the social worker as "scientist-practitioner" (see previous chapter) but its implicit assumptions apply equally well to EBP. Contrasting the definition of PBR that we provided earlier in this chapter we see that RBP like EBP requires that practice is driven primarily by research considerations whereby PBR seeks to introduce research into practice in ways that accommodate to pre-existing practice considerations, values, ethics, etc. In some sense, however, both may be seen as "evidence-based" but PBR relies on "practice-based" evidence generated within the practitioner's current practice whereby EBP relies on "research-based" evidence generated outside usually by other researchers.

Still, for our purposes, it is useful to detail the distinguishing differences between PBR and EBP. Box 1.1 does that.

Box 1.1 begins with a fundamental difference between these two approaches. PBR starts with practice considerations and what is referred to as "practice wisdom" which is the accumulated knowledge that practitioners gain from other practitioners, from their supervisors, from agency traditions and from their own "trial and error" experience. PBR both honors practice wisdom and considers it fallible. In other words, in PBR research can be used to test practice wisdom just as it can be used to test a research-based hypothesis. And while we don't begin by assuming practice wisdom is inherently flawed, we insist that when the practice-based evidence doesn't support practice wisdom then the practitioner must consider why and be open to change.

BOX 1.1   HOW DOES PBR DIFFER FROM EVIDENCE-BASED PRACTICE (EBP)?

PBR	EBP
Practice wisdom (inductive)	Prior research (deductive)
Rejects RCTs	Privileges RCTs
Qualitative and quantitative methods	Standard qualitative methods
Formative	Summative
Practice-driven by practitioners	Research-driven by academics

The starting point for EBP is prior research. EBP research texts begin by teaching practitioners how to systematically access and be critical consumers of published research conducted by others. In so doing, they emphasize the importance of "peer-reviewed" journal articles. In this book, as we indicated earlier, we value the contribution of prior research but it is not our starting point. Practice is our point of departure.

A second difference between PBR and EBP is that PBR rejects randomized controlled trials (RCTs) as an option for practitioners in most practice contexts whereas EBP "privileges" RCTs as the highest form of social work knowledge. And while some equally serious researchers have acknowledged the limitations of RCTs from a practice-knowledge generating point of view (Howe, 2004; Berk, 2005; Beutler, 2009; Nevo and Slonim-Nevo, 2011), PBR rejects them from a practice standpoint on ethical grounds.

Supporting the privileging of RCTs by EBP advocates is what is frequently referred to as the "hierarchy of evidence" (Roberts and Yeager, 2004). This hierarchical ranking of the credibility of evidence, which is basic to EBP places RCTs at the top and case studies employing non-statistical forms of research at the bottom. But not only is non-statistical qualitative research increasingly important in social work (Saini and Shlonsky, in press), but qualitative "case studies" of individual clients, client groups or programs are often legitimately and effectively used in social work training and supervision. In addition, many peer-reviewed practice journals rely heavily on evidence drawn from case studies in passing on valuable knowledge to their social work readership.

In that regard, PBR is "methodologically pluralist" (Epstein, 2009) by which we mean that we recognize the strengths and limitations of every research and knowledge-generating approach. And while we reject the uses of RCTs in most practice situations, we rely on the cause–effect logic of RCTs in those quasi-experimental studies that are ethically acceptable to practitioners. (We explain RCTs and quasi-experimental designs further in Chapter 4.)

In addition, we value equally qualitative research and forms of information generation that are natural to practitioners such as individual interviews, observations, group discussions, etc. By contrast, EBP gives exclusive attention to "research-based evidence" that comes from original data collection via "standardized" research instruments that have been developed by researchers to assess client problems, monitor interventions and evaluate outcomes. But while we recognize the usefulness of "universal" measures of practice, PBR provides a place for practitioner-generated measures that are less intrusive and burdensome and fit more comfortably in the practice context than do many standardized instruments. In fact, Epstein has argued quite extensively for the use of routinely available data in PBR. He refers to this form of research as "clinical data-mining" (CDM) (Epstein, 2010).

At the heart of the foregoing difference between PBR and EBP is an oft-used distinction between formative and summative research (Scriven, 1995). The former – central to the purpose of PBR – involves an emphasis on the immediate contribution of research to the practice context in which the research is being done. It recognizes that the practitioner's first priority is the practice context and client base with which she or he works. The practitioner is less concerned with proving that an intervention has any effect (the primary concern of EBP advocates) than with improving the service provided. Understandably, most academic researchers and EBP advocates are focused on summative research that allows one to make research-based generalizations beyond the context in which the research is conducted. This is why they favor RCTs and emphasize standardized quantitative measures.

Ironically, however, some have appropriately questioned the generalizability of RCT knowledge to more complex practice contexts than RCTs allow and to different client populations than those on which they were conducted (Aisenberg, 2008). Still, in EBP circles the familiar pyramid with RCTs at the top and qualitative case studies at the bottom remains the picture of the temple of evidence-based wisdom. For this EBP pyramid (see Figure 1.1), Epstein (2009) has suggested substitution of a non-hierarchical "wheel of evidence" (see Figure 1.2) in which all forms of research are valued and appreciated for their strengths as well as their limitations. That is the essence of "methodological pluralism".

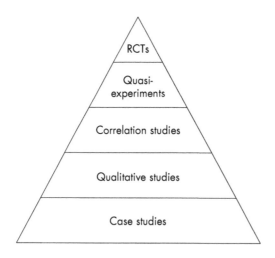

FIGURE 1.1   Hierarchy of evidence

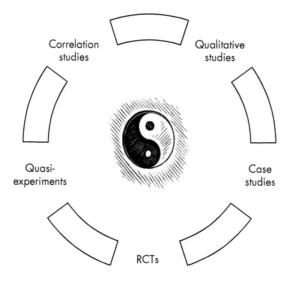

FIGURE 1.2   Wheel of evidence

In addition to its more open and flexible approach to research Figure 1.2 is intended to show how one form of research can generate another form. Hence CDMs which rely on retrospective studies using available data may lead to prospective quasi-experiments. These may, under particular conditions, lead to RCTs which, in turn may suggest the importance of a qualitative study to understand the "lived experience" of clients who received an intervention of one kind or another or to explain why an intervention might have worked or not (Saini and Shlonsky, in press).

Finally and ultimately, while PBR often is collaborative and involves research consultation, Box 1.1 clearly indicates that in PBR the practitioner and practice considerations prevail whenever there is a conflict between research principles and practice requirements. By contrast, in EBP studies as in all RCTs, research considerations come first. Thus if a client is in need of an intervention but is slated for the control group, or the "baseline" requirements of a single-subject design (SSD) study that requires a five-session assessment prior to "intervention", then practitioner advocacy for a departure from the research protocol is unlikely to be honored. Rather, the client is likely to be greeted with explanations about why the study will be compromised by providing an intervention during the control phase in the RCT or providing an intervention "prematurely" in the SSD.

Here again, we emphasize the PBR principle that places practice considerations above research when they come into conflict. That conflict is not inevitable, particularly when one is methodologically flexible. However, when it does occur, we are clear about our commitments.

In our final chapter, once you have developed more fully your PBR repertoire of practice-research skills and knowledge, we will offer a more complex and highly refined model of practitioner–researcher collaboration that is intended to empower practitioners in their dealings with researchers. Perhaps it's better to not empower you too much until the end of your research course however.

STRENGTHS AND LIMITATIONS OF PBR

Like any other approach to practice–research integration, PBR has its strengths as well as its limitations. These are identified in Box 1.2. Among its strengths is PBR's flexibility both in terms of the methods it employs and the subjects that it addresses. Thus, PBR is equally suited to assessing client and community needs as it is to documenting the quantity and quality of interventions and measuring clinical and programmatic outcomes. This will become apparent to you as you read about PBR study possibilities throughout this book and consider the PBR possibilities in your agency work.

A second strength of PBR is its compatibility with practitioner values and norms. While it may offer evidence that appropriately challenges "practice wisdom", it never challenges the legitimacy of the ethical principles and value commitments that you bring to your work. Instead, it finds ways to incorporate those values into your research.

Another strength of PBR is its low cost. None of the studies described in this book, nor indeed of the host of PBR studies that we have consulted upon, have required large research grants to conduct. Some consider this a limitation. However, since many of the agencies that employ social workers are strapped for financial resources and treat practitioner-research as a "luxury item" it is a significant strength that PBR can be

BOX 1.2   STRENGTHS OF PBR

- Flexibility
- Compatibility
- Cost
- Applicability
- Benefits to practitioners
- Benefits to clients

done relatively inexpensively. Most of all, what is required is practitioner motivation and confidence in her or his capacity to do it.

Once practitioners successfully engage in PBR it has all sorts of "secondary" benefits. Remarkably, despite all the anti-research sentiments described in the "reluctance" writing, we have found that practitioners who engage in PBR find it "replenishing" and a valuable opportunity to stand back and reflect on their work from a new perspective. Many have presented the results of their studies at professional conferences (in some terrific places) and some have published in peer-reviewed journals. Consequently, it would be incorrect to assume that because a PBR study originated as a piece of formative research that it has nothing to say of interest to practitioners in other comparable settings. Hence they may have summative implications. One of the most gratifying aspects of providing PBR consultation to practitioners is seeing the pride in professionalism that comes about as a result of publication or conference presentation or even presentation of findings within one's own agency.

Another benefit of PBR is that since it begins so close to practice, findings generated in PBR studies have direct application to practice. In fact, questions about how the findings might be used often motivate the study in the first place. This is not to say that unanticipated findings don't occur. However, application and utilization are among the highest priorities in PBR. This can only improve the effectiveness and efficiency of the work with our clients (as in quantitative studies) as well as the empathic understanding of our clients' lived experience (as in qualitative studies). The latter often give "voice" to individuals and groups that are otherwise "voiceless" by virtue of their status as service recipients. Some approaches to PBR – such as participatory action research – even include clients in the conduct, interpretation and dissemination of research. In other, less participatory forms of PBR, emphasis is still given to the question of how will this best serve the clients' interests. It is never research for its own sake.

That's the good news. We feel duty-bound to acknowledge the not-so-good news (see Box 1.3). As we've already indicated, PBR is not considered "gold standard" research among most researchers and research funders. In truth, "gold standard" RCTs are the best tools we have for demonstrating cause–effect relationships between social work interventions and outcomes, and for "proving" that what we did made a difference. Likewise PBR studies don't lend themselves as readily to summative generalization. As indicated above, sometimes they do. But more likely, PBR study findings are primarily used locally in the practice context within which they were done.

BOX 1.3   LIMITATIONS OF PBR

- Not "gold standard"
- Less generalizable
- Less fundable
- Less publishable

Though we recognize that social work is under pressure to demonstrate its effectiveness, as PBR researchers we are not willing to pay the ethical or professional price for that kind of definitive proof. Instead, we settle for less-than "gold standard" evidence. And it is striking how often well-conducted PBR research once presented makes a desired impact despite its methodological imperfections.

But for that, we must acknowledge another kind of price. PBR studies have been less fundable to date, because they carry the stigma of not being "gold standard" enough. Unfortunately, this has real consequences for practice-based researchers like us. Ironically, even if fundable, the low cost of PBR studies makes them unattractive to research academics who like large research grants, and to academic administrators who can legitimately use a certain percentage of every research grant for other organizational purposes such as photocopying machines or clerical staff.

Finally, although there are exceptions, PBR studies are (for now) less publishable in peer-reviewed research journals. But we can always learn from constructive criticism, so learn from the rejections, improve the paper, and then send it to a practice-oriented journal that will value it all the more.

SUMMARY OF KEY CONCEPTS

In concluding this chapter, let's summarize the main points that we wanted to convey to you about PBR. First that PBR begins with practice questions and practice wisdom and ends with practice applications. Second, that PBR is a collaborative process in which practitioners and researchers can be co-contributors to knowledge. However, when there are conflicts between the two perspectives, practice considerations prevail. Third, PBR is methodologically-pluralist and flexible. While RCTs are usually excluded from the repertoire, RCT logic is not. In addition, PBR studies can be retrospective or prospective; they can employ available or original data; they can be qualitative or quantitative; they can be descriptive or quasi-experimental: and they can even mix methods. Does that give you enough possibilities to work with? They can even begin as formative, inching their way to the summative though never quite getting there.

While we've discussed the differences between PBR and EBP at length we want to underscore the fact that they needn't be treated as though these differences are irreconcilable (Epstein, 2009). There's too much good social work research to be done to be wasting time carping about whose research is superior.

In the next chapter, we happily leave the "paradigm wars" behind and consider how to identify a researchable PBR problem.

Part 2

Engaging in the PBR process

Chapter 2

Establishing the practice-research problem

Purpose

This chapter illustrates how researchable questions emerge and evolve in the PBR process. It will help you identify practice-based and practice-relevant problems to explore using PBR. Therefore, the purpose of this chapter is to illustrate how research questions emerge in the PBR process; consider where questions may emerge from; and explore how practice problems are refined to become researchable questions, the answers to which can build knowledge for practice, theory or policy development.

INTRODUCTION

Do you ever wonder why some of your clients fully engage in treatment while others disappear after only one or two sessions? Do you wonder whether your program is effective in meeting its goals or even what the specific outcomes are that it is supposed to be achieving? Do you ever wonder what are the most common presenting problems in your caseload, and whether there are demographic differences in presenting problems? Do you wonder what the characteristics are of the youth who get a job at the end of your job-training program and those who don't? Or why some hospital ethics committees include social workers and others don't? Do you wonder whether the problems identified by the client on the intake form match the presenting problem identified by the social worker during their assessment? And do you ever wonder whether you and your colleagues are working similarly with agency clients and whether you are conducting your practice in ways that are consistent with what you are theoretically or programmatically supposed to be providing? If any of these questions ring a bell, then you have the beginnings of a PBR study.

PBR involves applying conventional research principles to questions that emerge from your direct contact with clients, your agency practice, and your participation in a professional community. The good news is that all of these examples are potentially researchable questions answerable by PBR studies that you and your colleagues can conduct.

Although some questions may be informed by prior research, the assumption made by evidence-based practice colleagues that a systematic and critical search of the research literature will answer these agency- and practice-specific questions is mistaken. Though it never hurts to see what others have found in other practice contexts, surmising that a particular approach to practice works everywhere (including your setting) with everyone (including your client base) is not a safe assumption. So while we devote a chapter to literature review (see Chapter 5), we see prior research efforts as potentially useful in other ways, e.g. providing research instruments, approaches to sampling, etc., but not necessarily to answer our specific practice question.

Within your own practice setting, the kinds of questions raised above can all be at least partially answered by PBR research studies that you can conduct. The results of these studies may not be conclusive and, if they are conducted correctly may actually lead to additional questions. In our opinion however, even these partial answers and the process of articulating the questions that inspired them are so much better than vague untested hunches and a pervasive feeling of "not-knowing" and not having the capacity to find out.

An important starting point in every PBR study is the identification of a problem that influences your practice in some way. Perhaps it is the felt need to affirm that you are doing a good job and that the interventions you are using are effective? Perhaps it is identifying differences in key characteristics of your clients and how they differentially engage with or react to treatment? Perhaps it's about better understanding the service needs of your client population? Problems may range from a very specific intervention question concerning the optimum length of a bereavement group to a more macro question concerning the implementation of new child welfare regulations.

The important and recurring theme here is that problem identification should emerge from practice and have the potential to impact your practice. In other words, no PBR study question starts with the phrase "Wouldn't it be interesting to know ..." That's because every PBR study is intended to inform practice decision-making. And while you don't know what you may find, you should have a clear sense of how you will use whatever you may find. On the other hand, the way your PBR study is like every other research study is that they are all conducted in a way that allows for you to discover something rather than to confirm your own biases. Hence, conducting a program evaluation that is designed to demonstrate only the good things about your program is PR (i.e. public relations) not PBR.

This chapter is designed to help you transform a general concern or question about your practice into a more specific, researchable question.

WHAT IS A PBR PROBLEM?

A problem, in general, can be defined as "any question or matter involving uncertainty, or difficulty" (*Random House College Dictionary*, 1980, p.1055), or "a question or puzzle that needs to be solved" (*Encarta world English computer-based dictionary*). An important aspect of these two definitions is the notion that we don't already know the solution, hence we need to work on solving the problem. Often, in social work practice we may think that we instinctively or intuitively know who our clients are, or what the most prominent presenting problems are, but sometimes what we think we know is not in fact the case. In fact, at the Adolescent Health Center at Mt Sinai Hospital in New York City, an entire collection of practitioner-conducted PBR studies was devoted to answering two very basic questions concerning young persons applying for health and mental health services at the agency, i.e. "What do kids want to talk about?" and "What do kids need to talk about?"

The answers to those questions, based on a differential analysis by gender, age and race of applicants were published in a book (Peake, Epstein and Medeiros, 2005) but more importantly, they were intended to inform and influence program planning and service provision. As research consultants to that project, both Dodd and Epstein can attest to the fact that those studies were conducted in such a way as to allow for findings that neither AHC practitioners nor research consultants anticipated. And, we hasten to add that their findings yielded many surprises, which were not in the least "intuitive". But that's why we do research of any kind, i.e. to fairly and objectively test our "gut feelings" rather than to simply support our biases. What makes PBR unique is that it is intended primarily to support the informational and decision-making needs of practitioners rather than to debunk what they do and what they know (Gambrill, 2010).

As with other personal service professions (Halmos, 1970), sometimes our perceptions of our clients and our practice are not accurate. As with other professions as well, we are human beings and subject to influences beyond our reflective capacities (Schon, 1983). In fact, in their list of the seven most common mistakes in starting research, Yegedis and Weinbach (2002) list "beginning by 'knowing' what will be found" (p.48) as number two. Given the danger of making assumptions about our practice and our clients, PBR is a good way to test our assumptions.

Number seven on their list is "failing to adequately define and specify the research problem" (Yegedis and Weinbach, 2002, p.48). So in the following sections we are going to explore ways to avoid these two common pitfalls.

WHAT IS PROBLEM FORMULATION?

In a seminal work written a half-century ago, the social work research pioneer Lillian Ripple (1960) wrote a chapter entitled "Problem identification and formulation" designed specifically for agency-based research. Reflecting on how practitioners experience their work, one of her key contributions was introducing the notion of a "felt difficulty", referring to those things that made practitioners feel unsure, uncertain or uneasy about what they do. Though the concept of PBR was not used in her day, her concept was as timely a half-century ago as it is today.

As a researcher, Ripple went on to suggest that identifying felt difficulties was a key part of the practice-relevant, problem formulation process. She proposed that before engaging in social work research of any kind, it is first necessary to determine whether:

1   a problem of concern to social workers exists;
2   whether additional knowledge is needed to solve the problem.

If the answer to both questions is "yes", then the task is to try to identify more specifically what key concepts are involved. In essence, she was urging us to try to be more specific about what we don't know!

Ripple's admonition is reflected in the beginning of every PBR consultation that we do. It's a lot like what you do when you first encounter a client or family or group or community. It involves a series of questions that further "specify" the presenting problem as well as any underlying problems. That specification is illustrated very directly in the aforementioned set of Mt Sinai adolescent PBR studies that distinguish between what new clients "want" and what they "need" (Peake, Epstein and Medeiros, 2005).

In that beginning step in the assessment as well as in the PBR process, you have to make sure that more than one outcome is possible and considered (otherwise, you may not need to do research because the results won't affect your action anyway). Similarly, as a clinician if your intervention approach is "one size fits all" then why bother doing an assessment?

Acknowledging the importance of Ripple's work, Sacks (1985) extended it by more fully exploring alternate ways in which research problems may be identified. He combined the four possible combinations of whether the problem was found either deliberately or accidentally with whether the researcher was cognitively prepared (understood the theories related to the topic) or not. He created a four-quadrant research model that he documented diagramatically. We have included a slightly modified version of his diagram here in Figure 2.1 adding the prevalence of the problem finding types within PBR and providing PBR examples of potential problems.

Quadrant I represents deliberate and focused problem finding with a prepared mind (i.e. theory-guided research). This quadrant represents theory-driven or theory-testing research, where a researcher with theoretical understanding of a particular issue purposefully sets out to test that theory in some way. This type of problem identification is less prevalent in PBR, but may be appropriate if, for example, you have received specific training on trauma-informed family treatment theory as well as practice and you would like to test the efficacy of that treatment against your current family treatment.

Quadrant II represents an "accidental" problem formulation interacting with a cognitively prepared mind. This refers to an unanticipated encounter with a phenomenon that you might recognize because you had prior training in practice or exposure to theory that unintentionally prepared you for recognizing and studying the problem (happy accidents). These occur in practice as well as in research when our theoretical training sensitizes us to recognize and identify particular patterns of behavior. The patterns of behavior may emerge in settings or populations that you don't expect, but you recognize them because the pattern is somewhat familiar to you.

Quadrant III refers to deliberate problem identification before the "researcher" has "an appropriate model to organize its exploration" (Sacks, 1985, p.220) (situation-dominated research). The researcher does not have a theoretical model to possibly

Prior cognitive preparation	Problem finding	
	Deliberate	**Accidental**
Yes	I Deliberate and focused theory-guided research Prepared minds selecting known problems Less prevalent in PBR e.g. Test the efficacy of a new theory-driven treatment against your current treatment	II Happy accidents Prepared minds encountering problems/new phenomena Less prevalent in PBR e.g. Recognize and study a familiar pattern of behavior in an unexpected client population
No	III Situation-dominated research Unprepared minds selecting known problems Very common in PBR e.g. Gathering systematic data about your practice context in order to generate a theoretical understanding	IV Off-the-map explorations (exploratory research) Unprepared minds encountering unexpected problems/new phenomena Occasional in PBR e.g. Encountering unexpected patterns of client behavior Gathering systematic data to develop a beginning understanding

FIGURE 2.1   Adaptation of Sacks' (1985) problem formulation model

describe or explain it, but does have an intimate familiarity with the situation that is being studied. This is the most common type of problem formulation in PBR studies. Often, as practitioner-researchers you have extensive exposure to the practice situation that you would like to study, but you do not yet have a framework for understanding it. You may have some hunches (what researchers would call "hypotheses") or think you see some regularities in the phenomenon (what researchers would call "descriptive theories") or thoughts about what causes it (what researchers would call "explanatory theories"), but you have never taken the time or made the effort to systematically state and test them. In this situation, the practitioner-researcher often seeks out existing theories that may appropriately fit the situation or develop a new theory from the systematic observations of the situation made by you and others implicated in the situation (what researchers would call "grounded-theory" development).

Quadrant IV refers to "off-the-map explorations", which occur when accidental problems are encountered by unprepared minds. In these situations you may encounter a new phenomenon at your agency that you are not familiar with, but that is intriguing and that you would like to know more about. In effect you are asking "what is going on here?" You do not have an organizing framework to work with so you begin to study the phenomenon and see what concepts start to emerge (this is what researchers call "exploratory research" and may include a grounded-theory approach).

As indicated earlier, within PBR much of our problem formulation occurs in quadrant III, but may occur in any of the four quadrants. The most important point to take from Sacks' (1985) model for PBR is that you don't have to be an expert in the theory or steeped in prior research literature to develop a researchable problem formulation, although you certainly can be. And, you do not have to set out to purposefully select a topic for research. Sometimes it selects you!

So, now you are thinking "OK, but how do I get started?" Well, the quick answer is "brainstorming".

Step 1: Brainstorming – so much to think about, so little time to think

In addition to being able to help people, one of the most exciting aspects of social work is that it is an expansive field with a range of practice arenas in which to work and populations with which to work. As a fellow social worker you will have the opportunity to serve and work alongside a diverse array of populations, in an equally diverse array of settings. You will also experience considerable variety of tasks within your particular position – some exciting and others less so.

Consequently, when launching a PBR project, any one social worker or set of social workers may have numerous areas of interest. For highly experienced practitioners who are new to PBR, the struggle is not coming up with a topic to study, but coming up with one – and only one – topic to study. In contrast, when faced with their first research assignment to "identify a problem", many novice social work students have been known to draw a complete blank. Whether overwhelmed or underwhelmed, this chapter can be equally helpful for those with too many ideas, as well as those with too few!

Whether working with others or alone, the brainstorming phase gives you an opportunity to write down, without editing yourself or your ideas, as many questions about your clients, your practice, your agency, or the policies that govern them as you can. You should jot down things that pop into your head as well as things that you have been thinking about in the back of your mind for a while. If you are having trouble coming up with any ideas, then begin to jot down areas or populations that are of interest to you. Perhaps you read an article for another class that you feel passionately about – does it involve a population, for example, children with autism, women with HIV, the severely and persistently mentally ill, or older adults with dementia? Or does it involve a topic – for example, ethical decision-making, therapist self-disclosure, cross-cultural family work? It may have involved a particular theory or model for practice, perhaps something as broad as group work or as specific as cognitive behavioral treatment for the depressed and homebound elderly. Brainstorming helps you to begin to get a list of possible problems down onto the page.

At this stage all you need to do is to identify the question, concern or need that you would like to learn more about in very broad terms that can be narrowed for PBR research purposes at a later point. The process involves being more sensitively attuned to your practice and being more quizzical about it than you have been in the past. This is done by observing patterns and themes that emerge within your practice from clients, at administrative meetings, or even within a community. This is one way in which PBR makes a contribution to practice even before the research has actually taken place. If you value self-reflection, PBR promotes it from the start.

Obviously, sometimes there is an "artificial" or imposed element to problem selection – particularly for students. For example, in research classes for social work programs, you as students are often asked to "do a research project" or at least to "develop a research proposal". Maybe that's when the "reluctance" mentioned in the introduction sets in (Epstein, 1987; Harder, 2010). More likely it's there from Day One. Both Epstein (1987) and Harder (2010) recognize the persistence of the pedagogical problem and offer different but related strategies to deal with it. Both involve encouraging students to conduct studies with available agency data. But more important, in so doing both ensure that student-conducted studies are practice-relevant.

So whether you follow Epstein's and Harder's research strategy or collect original data or both, what is most important in PBR is that the problem formulation emerges from practice, even if it is forced to emerge by yet another research professor asking for an assignment to be completed. Similarly, in practice contexts the research project may emerge because of outside forces, such as a funder requiring a program evaluation or an organization's board requesting a needs assessment. Even in these instances it is important that practitioners make sure they spend time refining and specifying the research problem so that it fully captures the concepts that are of concern and addresses the question that the funders, the board (and you) are most interested in.

Once you have your list of potential areas of enquiry, then individually or as a department, or team if this is a group effort, rank order the issues into the most important or most pressing concerns. Create a second list rank ordered for those that are of the most interest to you. Now look for issues that are high on both lists. In an ideal world your most pressing issue and the one of most interest to you would overlap at the top of both lists. Enquiring minds want to know, but they often want to know different things. In reality, however, it's not a good idea to let others totally define what you will study. Alternatively, as we indicated earlier, it's not a good idea to conduct a study that is based entirely on what would be "interesting" to you.

In the former instance, if you aren't passionately committed to the topic, then the chances of the study actually reaching completion are far more limited, especially as you juggle research tasks with an already full caseload. On the other hand, if you are too passionately involved in the area and think of PBR as a device to simply "prove" that you were right in the first place, think again. The great Roman historian Tacitus criticized prior historians for their failure to conduct research on the history of the Roman empire *sine ire et studio*, which if you didn't take Latin in high school, roughly translates as "without hate and zealousness". In less elegant words, they had axes to grind that tinted their research lens. Tacitus's counsel is as good in the 21st century as it was in the first.

Of course, if you have to complete your research assignment to get a grade towards graduation in the 21st century, then that may serve as motivation enough. But if you want it to really mean something for you, your agency and the people you both serve, then heed Tacitus. He won't be on the licensing exam, but his advice holds good for your practice as well as your research.

Step 2: Think through the relevance and impact

When considering a topic it is always important to ask "why do we care?" How many people are affected, in what ways are they affected, what would a change resulting from your findings mean for you, your agency, your clients or the community? As we said in Chapter 1, there should be an explicit, practice-based reason for conducting the research as well as some beginning notions about how the information will be used in practice. Try to think through whether or not the findings from your study have the potential to impact upon practice or policy decision-making, and the differential impact that alternative findings might have. But don't go too far thinking that you know what the findings will be because then you will be "reluctant" to learn from and use unanticipated findings that may arise.

Though it was not a PBR study, for his PhD research in sociology, Epstein was persuaded that professionalization was associated with social worker rejection of political activism and had a theory to back it up (clearly in Quadrant I according to Sacks). Despite his convictions, he conducted his study and constructed his survey instrument in such a way that he could discover that he was wrong. And he did just that. After the shock wore off, he further analyzed the data collected and learned a great deal about what he didn't know before but thought he did (Epstein and Conrad, 1978). That study was conducted so it could also be replicated, which it was 15 years later, by another PhD student. This later study (Reeser and Epstein, 1990) looked at whether historical changes in social work and in society had influenced the relationship between social worker professionalization and activism.

That is how research-based knowledge is accumulated. In PBR, replication and comparison are less likely to occur because, as we said in the previous chapter, its purpose is formative rather than summative (Scriven, 1995). Your PBR purpose is to inform practice decision-making rather than to make broad statements about the profession. But it is similar in the value that it gives to the importance of conducting research in such a way that you can discover that you are wrong as well as finding out things that you never even imagined or thought about. Also, both kinds of studies are "evidence-based". However in the study of social worker activism, the evidence was "research-based". In PBR studies, the evidence is "practice-based" and directly linked to practice.

Once you have made and compared your lists of possible topics, narrow down your focus to an area that seems like it will work for you. Try to choose something that is both interesting to you and where the findings have the potential to impact your practice in some way. (If you are still blanking on ideas then look at Table 2.1 for some examples of actual social work students' projects.)

Step 3: Narrower still – identifying key concepts

The next step in the problem formulation process is to identify the key concepts of concern within your problem area. The primary task here is to break down (researchers would say "deconstruct") your area of concern. You should begin to identify and define key concepts. So if we take the second example from Table 2.1 – adoptive parent–child attachment – the student first had to develop a nominal definition in words as in a dictionary definition to describe what she meant by "parent–child attachment". Then, since she was appropriately concerned with trying to strengthen the parent–child attachment, she had to come up with a measure of parent–child attachment. Researchers refer to the way we measure a concept as its operational definition (for more on concept measurement see Chapter 8).

Whether she was studying this through her own observations of mother–child relations, paper and pencil tests completed by the mother before and after completion

TABLE 2.1   MSW students' practice-based research projects

Problem area identified	Actual study question	Potential impact area
High infant mortality rates in Brooklyn	What are the attitudes and awareness of prenatal women towards infant mortality?	**Practice:** develop a program of education and outreach for prenatal women
Adoptive parent–child attachment	Is a parenting class intervention effective in strengthening adoptive parent–child attachment?	**Practice:** implementation of parenting class **Policy:** legislate funding for parenting classes to support adoptive parent–child attachment classes
Potential impact of art therapy on children living in domestic violence shelters	Do art interventions impact the social adjustment of children in two domestic violence shelters?	**Practice:** increase number of arts-based programs available in DV shelters **Policy:** increase funding for art-based support services for children living in DV shelters
The impact of health insurance coverage on stroke patients	Do stroke patients with HMOs receive comparable services to those with Medicare or non-HMO coverage?	**Policy:** require changes in HMO coverage for stroke patients
Self-disclosure regarding sexual orientation	What are the attitudes and practices of social workers related to sexual orientation?	**Practice:** in-service training related to sexual orientation and self-disclosure
Secondary trauma in post-9/11 disaster relief workers	What are the secondary traumatic stress levels among long-term disaster relief workers of the World Trade Center disaster of September 11, 2001?	**Practice:** provision of supports to reduce secondary trauma

of the training course, or by interviewing mothers who had taken the course or any other PBR strategy, she would have to come up with operational definitions of all of her key concepts. Since she chose to conduct a qualitative study of the mothers' experience of the course and its impact, she had to frame the questions she would ask and accompanying "probes" to be sure that the data she collected was honest, rich and not designed to either please or get rid of her. The final stage in the definitional process is specifying the intervention that she was testing, so that it was clear exactly what she was talking about. In other words, if she asked mothers about the "parenting program" in general, would mothers understand that she meant the classroom training they received rather than advice they received from caseworkers, other agency staff or even other adoptive parents? If she was interested in these, she would have to have separate questions and probes about each.

Once your area of interest is established then the specific research question(s) must be determined – both an overarching question and very specific sub-questions to bring your area of interest into a sharper focus. In the example, the over-arching research question was "Is a parenting class effective in strengthening adoptive parent–child attachment?" Some of the sub-questions were "Is there a difference in effectiveness for those parents who attend all ten sessions and those who attend less than five?" "Are there other differences between those who attend ten sessions and five sessions?" and "Is there a gender difference in the perceived impact of the training program?" If the student had been interested in the age, race or ethnicity of the parents to see if that impacted the effectiveness of the training, then she would have to be sure that she had access to that information either through case records, observation or direct questioning.

Step 4: Keeping your focus – staying on track

As we move through the steps in the problem formulation process, it is not uncommon to get pulled off course by other things in your work, school and personal lives. So, as you develop your study try not to make the common mistake of starting with a researchable problem and ending up with a study that looks at something else entirely. Continually return to your study's purpose and see how your questions and the data might continue to match your original concern to make sure that they mesh in the way that you want them to.

In addition, there is a necessary inter-relationship between the problem formulation and the study design selection. Within design selection (see Chapter 4) you will see that several factors influence your design choice, including time, money, and practice imperatives. As you make design decisions with consideration to these factors, it is important to pay continual attention to the original purpose of your study, and your problem formulation, so that the choices you make don't pull you away from addressing your original questions and the "felt difficulty" that concerned you when you started the process.

UNITS OF ANALYSIS

As you refine your problem, and develop your questions, you begin to determine who or what you want to study. In research terms this is referred to as your unit of analysis. The unit of analysis in a PBR study might be individuals, groups, programs, organizations, communities, or social artifacts. If you are interested for example, in how many and what types of people attend senior centers (i.e therapeutic day centers) in New York City, then we would count the individuals attending senior centers and try to determine something about their characteristics, perhaps their age, ethnicity, gender, physical ability, etc. The unit of analysis in this case would be the individuals within a specified age group who attend specified programs.

However, if you were interested in how many and what types of senior centers there are in New York City, then your unit of analysis would be senior centers in New York City and you would still have to specify what you meant by those terms. Once specified in a manner that makes most sense to you and others who would be interested in your findings, you might look at whether they are public or private and you may even map them geographically across the city. However complex your analysis becomes, your unit of analysis would remain senior centers in New York City. Hence, the unit of analysis represents the level that you are gathering data from or about. The unit of analysis could even be embedded in documents such as minutes of board meetings or client case records. In the former, the unit of analysis would be meetings and in the latter individual practice sessions.

COMPARING PROBLEM FORMULATION IN PBR TO A MORE "TRADITIONAL" RBP MODEL

In more "traditional" research-based studies, the problem formulation process (which looks a little like a funnel – broad at the top getting narrower at the bottom) begins with a broad identification of the felt need or problem. This problem is then refined into a more specific researchable problem through a process of thinking, some beginning reading on the topic, and perhaps initial conversations with experts. Once the specific researchable problem has been identified, research questions are formulated and a literature review is conducted. Through the literature review key concepts are identified, defined and operationalized until either a single hypothesis or a set of hypotheses emerges in quantitative studies or a focused research question emerges in qualitative studies.

In PBR the problem formulation process includes many of the same elements but they occur in a different order. The funnel may start in the same way with a broad identification of an area of interest. Or it may be reversed and begin from the narrow end of the funnel with a very specific question or concern. Either way, at some point you need to stand back and reflect on the issue from a broader perspective yourself and with practitioner colleagues and, in some cases with a collaborative research consultant or with your research professor. The interest area is similarly developed through personal reflection on the topic through internal dialogue and through dialogue with colleagues. This exploration process will help you develop clarity about what concepts are involved in the issue and what aspects of these concepts you are interested in. From there you begin to develop your nominal and operational definitions. And then you shape the question that you want to explore. Following this process helps you consider different ways in which you might approach answering your question, and before even thinking about collecting original data, consider what data may already be available to answer your question.

SUMMARY OF KEY CONCEPTS

In this chapter we discussed the problem identification phase, which is crucial in the research process since "if we can clearly identify what our problem is, we have taken a major step towards its solution" (Bloom, Fischer and Orme, 1995, p.63). We suggest that it is essential to spend time brainstorming around the area(s) that you have questions about. Then you can really narrow your focus, "drilling down" to the specific concepts that are of interest or concern to you or your agency. Just as when you are working with a client you begin by assessing the general area of concern before determining more specific notions of their presenting problems. So, in PBR you start with a vague sense of the problem area that you will ultimately focus on then refine your thinking to narrow the problem down into the particular aspect(s) that you are interested in. We describe how you think through the relevance of the findings in relation to your practice, develop nominal and operational definitions as needed, and then refine your question, including identifying your unit of analysis.

In many ways we should say that the problem formulation continues to be refined all the way through selection of a design, data-gathering methods, and selecting a sample. Often ethical and practical considerations such as time, money and access will importantly influence what you can study. Before proceeding any further, be sure you understand the concepts that make up your question (and therefore your study), that you are clear about their definition, and that you continually check that your focus has not drifted from your original intention as you move through the formulation and design process.

Chapter 3

PBR study purposes

Purpose

Different research studies, whether research-based or practice-based, have different purposes. This chapter describes and illustrates various PBR research purposes and offers guidance on how to select from among the PBR research designs that will be discussed in Chapter 4. After problem formulation, decisions about the purpose of your PBR study and your design strategy are the next important steps in your practice–research integration journey. Hence, this chapter is about choosing a PBR destination and the next is about choosing a PBR route to get there.

INTRODUCTION

Although "research-reluctant" students and practitioners may think that there is only one kind of research (and it's best left to the researchers), research-based studies have different purposes. So do practice-based ones. This chapter describes the differences within and between RBP and PBR studies. Then it shows how as a practitioner-researcher you can make informed choices about the purpose of your PBR study. Once that is done, the following chapter will show you how you can select from among various possible research designs. Needless to say, the two sets of decisions need to be integrated and, at the same time, compatible with practice considerations. It may sound complicated, but once you know the options it's not so hard.

In other words, this chapter is about naming your PBR study destination and the next is about the "road-map" for getting there. Subsequent chapters will be about "stops along the way" where decisions about sampling, data gathering, analysis, etc. will have to be made. And, whether you are driving alone, taking other practitioners, or even taking a researcher along for the ride, you can make informed choices about study purposes and research designs that will be most compatible with:

1   the knowledge-generating purposes of your study;
2   the practice setting within which the study is being conducted;
3   your provision of needed services to consumers.

Together this chapter and the next are based on the assumption that full and complete understanding of various possible research purposes and design options provide you, the practitioner-researcher, with all the information necessary to make informed decisions about your research without sacrificing practice principles and priorities.

Historically, research in practice settings has been conducted by academic researchers who have defined problems, chosen purposes and selected designs that privilege their research agendas at the expense of existing practice protocols, practitioner priorities and possibly even patient or client needs. For example, in an experimental study on the effects of social work services to "end-stage" renal dialysis (ESRD) patients, Beder (2008) set out to definitively demonstrate the effect of social work services on dialysis patients' depression and adjustment to their illnesses. Not a bad purpose.

However in order to achieve this purpose, Beder (2008) chose an experimental design in which patients were randomly assigned to practitioners who were instructed to provide either a minimal intervention (receipt of an informational pamphlet) to patients assigned to the "control group" or an "enriched" intervention involving multiple visits and psycho-social services to patients assigned to the "experimental group". For research purposes, which service package ESRD patients received was essentially a flip of a coin. Heads you get a full complement of services: tails you get a pamphlet.

While we asked you to stay open-minded about your study findings, in this case there was no surprise which group did better. In the process of reporting this important finding, the researcher made no comment about the possible denial of a more full complement of services to desperately needy end-stage patients who came up "tails". Similarly, there was no discussion of the wastefulness of providing extensive services to patients who were already doing well but came up "heads". Neither was there any discussion of what it must have been like for the social workers enlisted in Beder's research project to be prevented (for research purposes) from providing additional services to patients who needed them but found themselves in the control group.

Though the author didn't discuss the ethical issues involved in implementing this agency-based study, we're confident that it was approved by a hospital Ethics Committee and very likely as well by a university-based Human Subjects Research Committee (see Chapter 10 for a fuller discussion of research ethics and institutional review boards). No doubt workers as well as patients were informed of the "scientific" reasons for choosing the experimental design and the importance of rigorously complying with the research protocol, etc.

Clearly, however, both the researcher and the committees that approved this study were guided by a different set of values from those to which most practitioners (and as well most patients) would subscribe. The priority for the researcher was scientifically "proving" that social work intervention with ESRD patients was effective. What renal dialysis social worker would object to that purpose? But the design chosen intentionally bypassed practice wisdom concerning who required more extensive intervention and who did not. Inevitably it denied necessary services during the study period to some patients who would otherwise have received more than an informational pamphlet about dialysis.

From an RBP standpoint, this study was a great success. Patients in the experimental group did much better on all outcomes measured (Beder, 2008), thereby "proving" that social work with ESRD patients made a difference.

From a PBR standpoint, however, the study was problematic because it compromised both practitioners' and patients' ethical and personal interests. If challenged about this many academic researchers would justify Beder's (2008) study by saying that the only way to definitively demonstrate social work's effectiveness is through randomized controlled experimental trials (RCTs). In so saying, they liken social work practice research to drug studies claiming that the intervention (in this case a full complement of services) might be more harmful than a placebo (in this case a pamphlet).

A fully research-informed ESRD practitioner (and patient) would have seen the flaw in this analogy. At issue more generally are research priorities. RBP is about "proving". PBR is about "improving" through research that neither compromises practitioner nor patient priorities. A PBR perspective on practice–research integration opposes changing practice in order to accommodate to research considerations. It offers no resistance however to changing practice (or maintaining it) as a result of research. In fact it encourages it.

In the ESRD example, practitioners who didn't know better assumed that, if they were to do research relevant to practice, this was how it had to be. This is a common myth, reinforced by many research academics. As a result, practitioners who are enlisted in agency-based research projects often end up feeling disempowered, that their practice wisdom is disregarded and that the interests of service recipients are subordinated to the search for academic knowledge (Epstein, 2009, 2010).

By contrast, PBR studies give highest priority to maintaining practice integrity. In the process, sound research principles are adapted to best fit the practice situation. To do this properly, however, it is necessary for you the practitioner-researcher to have a comprehensive understanding of all aspects of the research process so you can make informed choices and "strategic compromises" at every stage of every PBR project you do. But if you think researchers in practice settings don't make similar compromises, you're wrong (Alexander and Solomon, 2006). It's just that they rarely write about them. Still, as PBR researchers, we can make good use of many sound research principles, practices and ways of thinking. We simply have to adjust them to the requisites of social work practice rather than the other way around.

STUDY PURPOSES: EXPLORATORY, DESCRIPTIVE OR EXPLANATORY?

Every PBR study involves a series of decisions about research methodology. The latter term refers to everything from problem formulation, study purpose, study design, type of data collected, sampling decisions, data-analytic decisions and finally, how to put the results back into practice.

Whether RBP or PBR, the basic decisions that every researcher must make concern:

1   the purpose of the study;
2   how to carry it out; and
3   how the resulting knowledge will be used.

These are the core questions of research methodology. But PBR is also about putting research back into practice, what we call research utilization. Though there may be unanticipated discoveries along the way, the intent of PBR is always to inform practice in the setting in which it was conducted – not conference presentations, not publications and not dissemination to other agencies. When those things happen (and they often do) it's even better. But the ultimate purpose of PBR remains better practice, programs and policies in the settings in which the studies are conducted.

Building on the "felt difficulty" and problem formulation from the previous chapter, this chapter is focused on the purpose of your study and the following chapter is about the logical structure for achieving that purpose, often referred to as the research design or the study design. In making decisions about purpose and design however, you must consider the study's intended use (Patton, 2008). Though purpose and design may vary, all PBR studies involve applied research. Whether they are at the clinical, supervisory, programmatic, administrative and/or community levels, applied research studies always emphasize practice applications.

As discussed in Chapter 2, self-reflective social workers of every type are interested in practice-based questions for many different reasons – knowing the purpose of your study helps you decide the best way to proceed and what kind of design to employ. Researchers usefully distinguish between three kinds of research study purposes:

1   exploratory studies;
2   descriptive studies;
3   explanatory studies.

Exploratory studies

Applied to PBR, the purpose of an exploratory study is to find things out about relatively new practice-relevant concepts or phenomena about which there is very little existing knowledge. Such topics might include newly emerging client needs, new practice concepts and/or relationships between client needs and practices not previously studied.

As you might expect, exploratory studies require more flexible designs and data-gathering techniques than do studies with other research purposes. Typically, they involve qualitative (non-numerical) rather than quantitative (numerical) methods of data gathering, and designs that can easily accommodate new practice terrain.

Conducting PBR studies at this stage of practice knowledge development, we simply don't know enough about what we are studying to be performing anything even approximating a research experiment, and there are practice contexts in which we may never think it appropriate to do so. Likewise, in exploratory studies we often employ sampling methods that are equally flexible, efficient and non-invasive. (Qualitative data gathering will be discussed more fully in Chapter 7 and PBR sampling in Chapter 9.)

The purpose of a PBR exploratory study is to get a beginning understanding of a practice-relevant issue, concept or set of relationships. Applied researchers especially PBR practitioner-researchers (like you) whose first priority is their practice are reluctant to invest a lot of time, energy and money into a project if you are not sure whether a phenomenon or relationship in question even exists or is relevant to practice decision-making.

Similarly, you would be unwilling to burden clients or consumers for research purposes even if the reason you are doing the research is ultimately to improve service. As a result, exploratory studies are often relatively small in scale and low in cost, time and effort to the pracitioner-researcher and in burden to the subject of research. Rather than to "prove" anything, exploratory studies are intended to provide information and sensitizing concepts that can then be studied further and more rigorously if appropriate at some later time. These smaller, shorter-term studies are sometimes referred to as "pilot studies".

Many PBR studies are exploratory in nature, arising from "felt difficulties" or questions social workers have about practice issues, concepts and/or patterns that they think may be emerging in their work. For example, a social worker working in a mental health program with adolescents may be interested in exploring ways in which social networking sites like Myspace and Facebook are affecting clients' feelings of social support or isolation. Alternatively, a health social worker working in a newly organized patient support program may be interested in knowing more about its impact on volunteers who are former cancer patients. Finally, practitioners in a social work unit may all be expected to use an innovative "strengths-based" approach that emphasizes client "resilience". An exploratory study might consider what sorts of client attitudes and behaviors social workers think represent indicators of this latter concept. Each of these studies can be conducted in multiple settings, with extensive data gathering from large populations using complex data-analytic techniques.

However, by conducting a pilot study in your own agency and simply asking clients, volunteers or practitioners a few well-chosen questions about their experiences and analyzing their answers relatively systematically, a practitioner-researcher can get at least the beginnings of an understanding of the issues. Thus, PBR emphasizes the importance of minimizing the burden of the study on potential respondents. Unlike some academic researchers, the PBR practitioner-researcher is always aware that research participation is a reciprocal process, so whether research subjects are consumers, volunteers or other practitioners, the burden of research participation on the subject should be minimized.

At the same time, that there may be a benefit to participating should not be overlooked. Occasionally, Ethics and Human Subjects Committees in universities are so wary of burdening research subjects that they fail to entertain this possibility. For example, clients may derive a significant clinical benefit from being asked about their life experiences, volunteers may derive greater self-esteem from being asked about their contributions to the program, and practitioners may derive a greater awareness about important practice concepts when they are asked to reflect upon them. More than one proposed research study has been rejected on grounds that the topic was "too sensitive" when it involved gathering information about something practitioners routinely discuss with clients, such as death or sexual behavior. (As noted earlier, more will be said about the ethics of PBR research in Chapter 10.)

Descriptive studies

Descriptive studies are those where the purpose of the study is to fully describe something that is relatively easy to identify but where some more systematic data gathering and a more complete description would help inform practice, program or policy. A non-clinical example of a descriptive study is the United States Census. Through the Census the US government is trying to describe the number and types of people living in households across the country, so that they are fully informed as they target resources and develop specific policies.

Descriptive studies concern themselves with what may seem like "mundane" details that are routinely recorded by practitioners, such as demographic characteristics, presenting problems, client strengths, or length of treatment. Nonetheless, these things are rarely studied and often empirically "unknown" to both practitioners and researchers. To researchers, they have little to contribute in and of themselves and only become interesting when correlated with other data, for example relationships between demographic characteristics.

Alternatively, practitioners may feel that they already have a "gut sense" or have derived "practice wisdom" about who they are serving and how, though they have never based their perception on a systematic inquiry. However in our individual and joint research consultations with practitioners in multiple settings, we have been struck by how frequently practitioners report surprise as a result of systematically describing who they are serving, what services they provide and what outcomes are achieved, even if they can't "prove" that it was their interventions that produced those outcomes. What is most important to them is simply knowing that improvements have resulted. In the Mt Sinai PBR studies focused on adolescent service applicants, it was less surprising that practitioners didn't know what client characteristics were associated with what service requests (Peake, Epstein and Medeiros, 2005).

Similarly, a descriptive study of the demographic characteristics of elderly residents in an assisted-living facility, the service requests that social workers received from them, the services they provided and to whom may seem obvious and pedestrian to an RBP researcher, but for a PBR practitioner-researcher the patterns described in such a study can reveal important, unmet service needs of residents and significant training gaps for workers.

Although they are relatively straightforward to conduct, gut feelings and practice wisdom aside, descriptive PBR studies often yield significant unanticipated findings, some positive and some less so. But that's why we do research.

While the examples given above are entirely quantitative, descriptive studies may also be qualitative and based on detailed descriptive accounts of intervention behavior based on direct observations, process recordings or indirect observations taken from case records. Cordero and Epstein (2005) used the latter approach to describe casework interventions employed in successful foster-care reunification cases. Though their study could not claim that it was these interventions that made the difference, it did demonstrate the challenges and complexity of reunification practice and the skill-repertoire required of social workers who do it. Though methodologically and conceptually simple, the value of qualitative and/or quantitative descriptive studies to the practitioner-researcher should never be underestimated.

Within the context of PBR, there are three types of descriptive studies that are especially valuable to practitioner-researchers (Epstein and Tripodi, 1978):

- needs studies;
- monitoring studies;
- outcome studies.

Needs studies

Often referred to as needs assessments (Royse *et al.*, 2009), needs studies describe the service requests and expectations as defined by consumers and their needs and or "risk factors" and strengths or "resiliency and recovery factors" (McCubbin, 1998) as defined by practitioners. As Peake, Epstein and Medeiros (2005) have shown, PBR researchers must always be careful not confuse client requests and worker perceptions of risk. Likewise, one should never assume that service applicants are solely described by risk profiles, neglecting to assess the strengths they bring to every problem situation (Saleeby, 2008).

Returning to the collection of descriptive needs studies of adolescent mental health applicants mentioned earlier, Peake, Epstein and Medeiros (2005) and the numerous PBR practitioner-researchers who contributed to their collection make an important distinction between the services that adolescents request (i.e., what they "want to talk about") and those that a mental health professional conducting an intake interview might discern (i.e., what they "need to talk about"). Likewise, in the self-administered intake instrument that all treatment applicants completed prior to seeing an intake worker, respondents were asked questions about their risk behaviors in multiple sectors of their lives but careful attention was also given to what they felt they did well.

Naturally, over the course of treatment, information about all of these may emerge and ideally change. However, in planning new programs or in making a treatment plan for an individual client, it is essential to keep in mind the distinction between client or community service requests or expectations and service needs that are identified by professionals. In PBR needs studies, both must be taken into account and neither should be considered of lesser importance.

Monitoring studies

Monitoring studies involve descriptions of social worker and/or program interventions. These may include everything from behavioral or psychotherapeutic interventions, advocacy efforts, provision of concrete services, referrals, the use of groups, organizing efforts and all the other ways in which social workers do what they do. Monitoring studies might be based on data in client records, accountability reports, time and activity studies, observations of practice or interviews with service recipients about the services they did receive.

A special type of monitoring research study is what researchers call fidelity studies. These studies consider how "faithfully" practitioners are adhering to a particular intervention approach. Thus, in a study of an Intensive Family Preservation (IFP) program, Hanssen and Epstein (2007) looked at the fit between case record data describing patterns of "actual" service provision and the "ideal" IFP model of program implementation.

While potentially very valuable, a frequent criticism of monitoring studies is that they tell us nothing directly about whether clinical or program outcomes are achieved. In other words, what is the relationship between social worker interventions and the results of these interventions?

Thus, number of "client contacts", individual or group sessions or community meetings and the numbers in attendance only document our efforts and whether the intended beneficiaries of our efforts show up. Nonetheless, monitoring studies can tell us very important things about what practices take place with whom and the quality and quantity of these practices. It's not the "whole story" but it's a very important part of the story. Elsewhere, Epstein (2010) refers to a family treatment training program for psychiatric residents provided by a prestigious family treatment training institute. A PBR monitoring study of the clinical sessions provided by these residents revealed that even after their training, the vast majority of their interviews involved individual family members rather than couples and/or their children. Though this study was extremely simple and efficient to carry out, admittedly it had nothing to say about the efficacy of their interventions. However, it was both surprising and valuable for the training program director to have conducted.

Still, it is correct to say that monitoring studies tell us little about the possible results of clinical, program or policy interventions. By contrast, the final type of descriptive study to be considered here – outcome studies – describe the extent to which intended clinical, programatic or social action purposes are realized. And, in doing so, outcome studies make an invaluable contribution to practitioner understanding.

Descriptive outcome studies

Descriptive PBR outcome studies focus on whether or not intended individual client, family, group, organizational and/or community objectives are actually achieved. Such studies may include everything from satisfaction surveys to recidivism and relapse studies and represent the essence of what is called evaluation research.

While for accountability purposes, considerable external pressures are placed on programs of all kinds to demonstrate with empirical evidence that they achieve the outcomes they are funded to achieve, every self-reflective social worker should want to know whether her or his efforts are yielding the benefits sought for clients and the community. Services and interventions are not ends-in-themselves; they are means to ends. For RBP researchers and EBP advocates, demonstrating the cause–effect linkage between interventions and outcomes is what evaluation research is all about. That's precisely why for them the RCT represents the "gold standard".

For PBR practitioner-researchers by contrast, descriptive outcome studies have great value for the practitioner-researcher though they do not assure us that when things improve, it is the result of our interventions. Even in "total institutions" (Goffman, 1961) such as prisons, mental hospitals and juvenile correctional institutions all sorts of planned and unplanned factors impinge on clients' lives (Polsky, 1977).

Additionally, clients have their own inner resources, which they can draw upon without our help. So while we might like to take credit for all positive client outcomes and blame other factors for the absence of positive change (and certainly negative outcomes), it is important to remember that descriptive studies of program outcomes say little about what determined them. Hence the PBR practitioner must recognize that "outcome-only" studies are exactly what they claim to be, that is to say they describe what happened, but they don't explain it. They say nothing directly about what caused those positive objectives to be achieved. Consequently, we must be very careful about inferring that, once documented, everything good is the result of our interventions and that the absence of positive change (or worse still, things worsening) is a consequence of things beyond our control. Nonetheless, in the absence of more sophisticated cause–effect studies (which as we saw in the ESRD study can have serious practice limitations), descriptive outcome study possibilities should be considered an option by every practitioner-researcher.

Some PBR descriptive studies may combine elements of needs studies, monitoring studies and/or outcome studies by collecting data relevant to more than one of these study purposes. However, what makes even those "descriptive" in character is that they do not look at interrelationships between needs, interventions and outcome data – taking each type of data by itself and documenting what we know about each. Moreover, they can be qualitative, quantitative or a mix of both. Even these combined study types are not as sophisticated or complex as studies that seek explanations for client outcomes, but they still tell us a great deal more than we knew before the study was done. And even the simplest descriptive outcome study can tell us what clients were like when they completed the program.

Explanatory studies

Explanatory studies, as you might expect, try to predict and explain things. As such, they require considerable prior knowledge about what one is doing and why. Additionally, they require highly structured experimental designs, highly refined standardized data-gathering instruments and complex data-analysis techniques to demonstrate that the relationships found are consistent with predictions made and to eliminate other possible explanations for why that is so. Beyond the repertoire of most practitioner-researchers, such studies (as we saw earlier) may also involve design elements and instrumentation that are objectionable to clients and/or practitioners (Epstein, 2001).

Still, it is essential for the PBR practitioner to understand the elements of experimental designs like RCTs because experimental logic is built into a variety of less rigorous, more flexible quasi-experimental designs that are more suitable to practice application.

Experimental and quasi-experimental studies might test the effectiveness of an intervention, asking for example, does a long-term support group for adolescents reduce their risky sexual behaviors and their illegal substance-use? They might also compare different treatments, asking whether a short-term psycho-education group is as effective as a long-term support group in reducing the risk behaviors of the adolescents. Or, they might ask, how do both of those interventions compare to no intervention at all? Experimental and quasi-experimental designs may also be used to look at the differential impact of treatments by gender or age or some other characteristic.

A major difference between experimental and quasi-experimental design types is that rigorously structured experimental studies are the closest we can come to "proving" the existence of a cause–effect relationship between an intervention that we employ and an outcome we seek to achieve, ruling out other possible explanations. By contrast, a quasi-experimental design only approximates that inference and leaves open other possible explanations. (More about design elements will be discussed in the following chapter.)

Given the realities and ethics of practice, however, in quantitative PBR studies quasi-experiments are probably the closest we can get to the "gold standard". This explains why Epstein's first paper on "mining" available clinical records is subtitled "Mining for silver while dreaming of gold" (Epstein, 2001). More recently, rethinking the "gold standard" ideal, he has suggested that in some respects, quasi-experimental studies generate more useful practice information than experiments because experiments intentionally minimize the effects of everything other than the intervention, whereas quasi-experiments may focus on ways in which different client groups respond to the same or different interventions regardless of what else may be going on (Epstein, 2010). Although they are less rigorous than RCTs from an RBP point of view, the information quasi-experiments generate may be of greater interest from a PBR point of view to practitioners than definitively proving that an intervention works for an unspecified general population. This is because in essence quasi-experiments study the person-in-environment, which is more consistent with social work values.

A challenge for the practitioner-researcher then, arises from wanting to conduct research that will inform practice without setting up artificial or possibly unethical situations in which consumers are denied the services they desire in order to satisfy research requirements. To meet this inherent conflict between research and practice requirements, "strategic compromises" are required that are informed by an understanding of experimental logic but allow more "natural" patterns of practice to prevail. Some of these strategic compromises involve design modifications – others statistical and data-analytic strategies.

In our advocacy of PBR, it would be foolish to assert that there is no conflict between practice and research or institutionalized conflicts between academic researchers and practitioners. RBP and its current EBP manifestation is one approach to "reconciling" these conflicts by encouraging or even restricting practitioners to use only those interventions which have been "proven" effective using "gold standard" research methods. This set of criteria tends to limit practitioners to interventions that lend themselves to RCTs (e.g. cognitive behavioral therapy – or CBT – approaches) and to a focus primarily on client problems that are amenable to behavioral interventions. Here, the danger is that the means become ends in themselves, and we neglect problems and interventions that don't fit the EBP prescription.

A recent survey of the use of "empirically-supported" and "non-empirically-supported" interventions showed (undoubtedly to the chagrin of the researchers who are EBP advocates) that social workers who used more of the former also used more of the latter (Pignotti and Thyer, 2009). The authors dismissively refer to the latter category of interventions as "NUTS" – an acronym for "novel, unsupported, therapeutic interventions" implying something about the users of these interventions. However rather than finding two types of clinicians, i.e. the evidence-based practitioners versus the "NUTS", what they found was practitioners who used a full repertoire of interventions (evidence-based and not) and those who used a relatively narrow range of interventions (similarly evidence-based and not).

The tensions between RBP and PBR are central to our decision-making about research purposes and designs. Our position however as PBR advocates is to be as "methodologically rigorous" as possible in seeking practice knowledge, without compromising the integrity of the practice. Once you decide on whether your PBR study is going to be a needs study, a monitoring study or an outcome study, your next step is to choose an appropriate study design.

When the purpose of the study and the design are experienced by the practitioner as being in conflict, then the PBR practitioner should always side with the practice purpose. Still, lots of useful design options remain. These design options and additional factors affecting the selection of the appropriate design for your PBR study will be presented in the next chapter.

SUMMARY OF KEY CONCEPTS

In this chapter we introduced the idea of exploratory, descriptive and explanatory studies. Most PBR studies are either exploratory or descriptive though some approximate explanatory studies. In addition, we discussed three different types of descriptive studies – needs studies, monitoring studies and outcome studies. Throughout the chapter we consider the compatibility between different research purposes and practice priorities. The PBR decision-making principle (that strategic compromise is used to ensure that practice integrity supersedes research priorities) is highlighted.

Chapter 4

PBR research designs

Purpose

Research design refers to the logical structure of your study. In any given study of practice, multiple design options are available. In PBR studies, however, the design chosen must "privilege" practice rather than research priorities and protocols. This chapter describes a range of PBR designs and the factors you should consider in choosing one.

INTRODUCTION

Now that you've formulated a practice-based problem you want to research and your study purpose has been determined, your next step is choosing a research design that suits your purpose, but does not compromise your practice. Here, as at other methodological decision-points in the PBR study process, "strategic compromises" are required. They make it possible for you to select practice-friendly research designs to answer practice-based questions and to generate knowledge that is directly applicable to your practice.

   This chapter discusses factors that you as a PBR practitioner-researcher have to consider when selecting a research design. Starting with "ideal" RBP design options, we move from experimental to quasi-experimental to descriptive PBR designs, considering their strengths and weaknesses in seeking a proper balance between design rigor (i.e. how certain you are that your results are accurate and caused by what you think they are) and practice integrity. Potential threats to the internal validity of various study designs are also discussed. Finally, both practice and practical (e.g. time, money, etc.) considerations are introduced into the decision-making process. In RBP as well as in PBR studies, practical considerations must be taken into account. However in PBR studies, issues of intrusiveness, disruption of practice protocols and burden on clients as well as on workers are of paramount concern.

Once a PBR design has been selected, you'll have to make a series of smaller decisions relating to the details of your design. In practice research of any kind, these rarely come down to right or wrong answers as much as different options that each have their unique knowledge-generating pros and cons. None are perfect. Each option leads to different information with different potential applications. Likewise, for each stop along the way smaller decisions influence and refine the larger decision about the overall research design for the study.

If you are driving solo, this means having a research-informed internal dialogue with yourself about the various options and considerations. Though you might prefer listening to your iPod, this can still be fun. If this is a team effort, turn the volume down since it means an active dialogue with PBR colleagues about the pros and cons of various design options. If you have a research consultant along for the ride, turn the music off completely because you'll want to be sure to be a full participant in the discussion, always keeping in mind the practice implications of design selection and implementation.

TAKING A CLOSER LOOK AT EXPERIMENTAL DESIGN

As we indicated in the previous chapter, explanatory studies *aka* experimental studies *aka* classical experiments *aka* RCTs (randomized controlled trials) try to determine the cause–effect relationship between different phenomena (or variables) and the explanation for that relationship. In the context of practice-research the "causes" or what researchers refer to as independent variables are usually interventions of some kind such as individual counseling, family therapy, participation in a mutual support group, community action, etc.

The "effects" or consequences in which practice researchers are generally interested are clinical or programmatic outcomes of some kind, e.g. decreased depression, increased family cohesion, improvement in self-esteem, reduction in community violence, etc. Researchers refer to these as dependent variables because, in these studies, the assumption implicit in the study or the hypothesis to be tested is that variations in the dependent variables are determined by variations in the independent variables. For example, if you are interested in studying the impact of a 16-week telephone support group on the level of isolation felt by seniors having chemotherapy treatment for cancer, then your dependent variable is social isolation and your independent variable is a 16-week telephone support group. Conceptually, we refer to this predicted co-variation as correlation, but in quantitative studies we also have statistical procedures for measuring it (we'll discuss those in Chapter 12).

In experimental practice-research designs, the independent variables (treatments) are intentionally manipulated by the researcher or the researcher's surrogate (e.g. the practitioner) in order to rigorously determine whether they have the desired effect on the dependent variables (depressive symptoms, family cohesion, etc.). More specifically,

the manipulation of the independent variable (IV) involves very deliberately monitoring access to, involvement in or receipt of interventions by participants as well as the
"dosage" received, i.e. frequency, intensity, and type of service. Those assigned to experience the intervention are referred to as the "experimental" or "intervention" group,
and those who do not receive the intervention are referred to as the control group. In
rigorously controlled experiments, special efforts are made to ensure that those in the
control group have no access to the experimental intervention either within the agency
context or anywhere else for that matter. In practice research studies where it is ethically
or legally untenable to deny service entirely, such as the end-stage renal dialysis (ESRD)
study discussed in Chapter 3, a control situation is created by providing a minimal or a
"traditional" or "treatment as usual" intervention (Beder, 2008).

As a critical consumer of information you are probably thinking, well, just because
two variables change in time together you can't conclude that one causes the other. So
for example, you may be thinking that if adolescent participants in a year-long, weekly,
school-based support group show improved self-esteem after they have completed the
program, it is quite possible that the explanation for this improvement has little or
nothing to do with group participation.

This is where the "R" in RCT comes into play. Randomization (also known as
random assignment) is a process by which every individual or unit of analysis has
an equal probability of being selected for the experimental or for the control group.
In RBP studies it involves seeing to it that assignment to the experimental or control
groups is based upon chance alone rather than any personal bias, client preference or
practitioner judgment about who is most in need, or will benefit most, or any other
such consideration. Random assignment is intended to answer your suspicions by
ruling out any other possible explanation or bias that might have caused the observed
change in the experimental group. Since any unexpected and unexplained changes in
one group could also reasonably be expected to occur in the other group, the intervention (the IV) is the only possible explanation for any change that occurred. In principle
then, the combined use of a control group, an experimental group and randomization
allows for a complete explanation of any significant differences that result between the
two groups.

Applying experimental logic to our mutual support group study means that those
who participate in the support group and those who do not are randomly chosen so
that other potential explanations, such as IQ, grade point average (GPA), gender, race,
social class, etc. are equally distributed in both groups. As a result, if group participants' self-esteem scores are significantly better than those measured in the control
group by the end of the year, then the only plausible explanation is that it was the
support group participation that made the difference.

On the other hand, if both groups improved equally, then we might infer that
maturation might have explained the change but we can be certain that it wasn't
explained by support group participation. If the support group participants had
lower self-esteem by the end of the year but were comparable to the control group
at the beginning, then it would imply that support group participation was somehow
damaging to their self-esteem. If neither group's self-esteem changed during the year,
this would strongly suggest that neither maturation nor support group participation
had any effect.

The powerful advantage of the RCT is that it allows us to consider and measure
all of these possibilities and more. In fact, when an RCT is combined with advanced

statistical procedures we can assess the effects of multiple variables together as well as partial explanations i.e. the amount of statistical contribution each makes to the overall outcome. So you can look at the impact of age, race, gender and socio-economic status as well as participation in the support group and understand the differential contribution of each.

Thus, if support group participation was found to significantly improve self-esteem and we had IQ scores for all participants, it would be possible to see whether those with higher IQs benefited more from support group participation and by how much. That is what we refer to as multi-variate analysis and will be discussed briefly in Chapter 12. For further reading on this topic, see also Weinbach and Grinnell (2010) *Statistics for Social Workers*, and Craft (1990) *Statistics and Data Analysis for Social Workers*.

For now, it is sufficient for you to know that RCTs employ randomization to rule out other possible explanations for intervention outcomes. This applies to explanations that you can think of, as well as those you can't possibly imagine.

VARIATIONS IN DESIGN

For reasons discussed in the previous chapter, "gold standard" RCTs do not lend themselves well to most practice situations. More specifically, random assignment conflicts directly with the value of differential assessment and varied intervention based upon it. Likewise, denial of an assumed more beneficial service necessary for creating a control group also does not sit well with social workers or their clients. In other words, in experimental studies the value researchers place on knowledge-generation often runs counter to the value practitioners give to service provision. Still, there exist a wide range of design variations that can be applied to practice-relevant research questions and used in PBR studies. We will explore these designs now as they neither require the withholding of services nor artificially assign clients to the services they receive.

The simplest design and the one most likely to be used by PBR researchers (and perhaps least favored by RBP researchers) is the "post-test" or "after-only" or "outcome-only" design (see Figure 4.1 on page 51) in which everyone eligible for a service receives it and outcome measures are taken upon completion of the service. Thus, you might survey homeless client risk behaviors after completion of a psycho-education group (about mental illness, psycho-pharmacological medication and illicit drug-taking) to determine their risk profiles and perhaps the demographic factors that are associated with variations in them. Such a descriptive study of what participants are like post-psycho-ed would have considerable value from the standpoint of telling you about remaining client risks and service needs and might suggest future refinements for the psycho-ed program and other kinds of service provision, but it would tell you nothing directly about the impact of your program. You might even ask them how participation in the program had affected their risk behaviors and how the program might be improved? Their responses would be quite valuable in themselves and clearly, such a design would be much less intrusive and problematic to practitioners than an RCT, but it would offer the least from the standpoint of causal knowledge-generation. It would provide no useful comparisons prior to group participation or with those who did not receive the intervention, nor would it rule out other possible explanations. Still, an after-only study tells you more about the achievement of clinical or programmatic or community interventions than no evaluation at all. "After-only" designs are probably used most frequently in PBR studies. However, for reasons that make them most acceptable to practitioners (i.e. they are not intrusive to practice) they are least acceptable to researchers (i.e. they are not explanatory).

Such a descriptive, non-explanatory design would be represented by the diagram in Figure 4.1.

As we discussed in the previous chapter, studies that utilize many of the principles of experimental studies but do not employ random assignment are known as quasi-experimental studies. Studies that use quasi-experimental design are more rigorous than post-test only studies but sit more easily with practitioners than RCTs as they can be conducted without the use of either randomization or the denial of treatment to anyone. So, for example, when conducting a quasi-experimental study with homeless, mentally ill individuals you may take a baseline measurement of risk behavior or pre-test to see how the group is doing before you start and then you run your treatment and then we see how they are doing afterwards by taking a post-test. A simple pre-test/post-test, sometimes called a Time1/Time2 or before/after study, like that can be drawn as a diagram by using O to represent something that is being observed or measured like risk behavior (e.g. taking illicit drugs, or going off prescription medications, etc.) as in our example, we then use an X in the diagram to represent the intervention that is being studied (a 10-week psycho-ed group) to see if it has an impact (post-test). That study could be drawn as in Figure 4.2.

To improve your confidence that the psycho-ed group explained any positive difference that you found after the 10-week period, you might take a series of baseline measures, prior to enrolling participants in the psycho-ed group so that you can be sure that the behaviors you observed before intervention were stable and not idiosyncratic or based on an effort to please or to ingratiate you the practitioner to provide more services. A diagram representing that experimental embellishment is represented in Figure 4.3.

It would be even better if you were able to determine whether the benefits observed immediately after completion of the psycho-ed program were sustained over time. In other words, if you could assess whether the value of the intervention program wore off. To look at this, you could add an additional observation period at some point after the post-test perhaps at 3, 6, 9 or 12 months after completion of the group. The embellished design would add one or more extra observation points and would look like Figure 4.4.

This design would let you see whether the reduced scores at post-test were maintained or whether risk behavior scores reverted to pre-group levels or even got worse. It would be possible to argue, however, that with such a vulnerable group as homeless, mentally ill substance abusers it would be necessary to follow up their behavior over a 12 month period, before you could safely infer that participation in the program had lasting effects.

How could you know whether these effects were the result of your psycho-ed program or simply due to the provision of stable housing? You can't answer that question without comparing an equivalent group of homeless, mentally ill substance abusers who did not receive a psycho-ed intervention. That would require use of a control group which in a "perfect" RCT would not only have to be compared with a group that received psycho-ed, but would have to be prevented from receiving any other kind of intervention. Only by doing this, could you infer that any positive benefits that were observed in the intervention group, but not in the control group, were the

X   O

Where:
X = Intervention (Psycho-ed group)
O = Observation (measurement of risk behaviors)

FIGURE 4.1   Post-test only design

O_1 X O_2

or   Risk behavior score (RBS)$_1$, Psycho-ed group   RBS$_2$

FIGURE 4.2   A pre-test/post-test design

O_1 O_2 O_3 X O_4

or

RBS$_1$ RBS$_2$ RBS$_3$ Psycho-ed group   RBS$_4$

FIGURE 4.3   Multiple baseline pre-test/post-test design

O_1 X O_2 O_3

or

RBS$_1$ Psycho-ed group   RBS$_2$ RBS$_3$

FIGURE 4.4   Pre-test/multiple post-test design

consequence of psycho-ed. And, in order to ensure the comparability of the two groups to begin with, participation in one or the other must have been based on a process of random assignment.

While RCTs are considered the "gold standard", additional embellishments are sometimes added to provide even greater assurance of causality than in the "classic" experimental design described earlier. These embellishments can be applied in PBR studies as well. In "true" experimental design, by virtue of randomization, the control group is assumed to be comparable to the intervention group in every way other than receipt of psycho-ed intervention. Of course, comparability could also be established by comparing the two groups on variables such as demographic characteristics, drug histories, work histories, etc. prior to intervention, just to be sure.

To fully implement the even more rigorous experimental design, both groups would be observed at three time points (at baseline, after 10 weeks, and at 12 months, which can also be stated as pre-test, post-test, and 12 months post-test). To maintain the design requirements of the RCT, they would receive no intervention other than

$$O_1 \quad X \quad O_2 \quad O_3$$
$$R$$
$$O_1 \qquad \quad O_2 \quad O_3$$
where R = randomization

FIGURE 4.5   Experimental design

the provision of housing, which everyone receives. Moreover, steps would be taken to ensure that they did not receive psycho-ed or any other supportive interventions elsewhere. So the diagram for this study would look like Figure 4.5.

In an even more refined RCT, you might go on and create a third, randomly assigned group that received no housing at all and were left on the streets during the period of the study. That way, you could definitively "prove" what kind of contribution your social work services made and determine how much the "housing alone" condition contributed to the outcomes observed.

But at this point, you are probably asking "Is it worth the price?" Clearly, as you ratchet up the research knowledge contribution of your study, you raise more practice and ethical issues about the costs to your own practice commitments and to your clients of generating such knowledge. As a PBR practitioner, the challenge is to learn as much as you can about the impact of your practice without compromising your own values or the interests of your clients or client community. Therein lies the "threat" of research to practice.

UNDERSTANDING CHALLENGES TO RESEARCH INTEGRITY

However, before considering how to deal strategically with that challenge, it's important for you to know more about the "threats" that RBP researchers worry about in maintaining the integrity and rigor of their RCT research designs. It is important for you to understand these "threats" since you will then understand the ways in which you need to be careful when making inferences from your findings and describing your study's limitations. So, for example, there may be something about those who participated in the psycho-ed group that made them different from those who did not. Perhaps, instead of random assignment, intake workers innocently and in a well-intentioned way assigned to the intervention group the people they thought would benefit most from psycho-ed because they were "high functioning" individuals. In this instance, one would very likely observe that psycho-ed participants fared better at the end of the study. However, their doing so could not be safely attributed to the psycho-ed intervention but rather to the superior strengths of those who were referred to it in the first place. Indeed, these individuals might have done better on their own simply because they received stable housing. Although this is what researchers would negatively label creaming, practitioners would positively view it as best practice – i.e. matching client to program so as to maximize the benefits of the program under conditions of resource scarcity. The problem from the standpoint of research knowledge generation is that we might infer that the program was making a positive difference when it was really only making a positive difference for a particular type of client.

Alternatively, intake workers might assign those clients to the intervention group who demonstrate the greatest need – i.e. those individuals with more severe symptoms, fewer resources, least compliant, most addicted, etc. The basis for this pattern of group assignment might justifiably be greatest need. Under these conditions, it would possible that those receiving the psycho-ed intervention seemed to fare worse than those in the control group when actually they were more troubled to begin with. The problem from the standpoint of research knowledge generation here is that we might infer that the program was making a negative difference when it really wasn't.

A third possibility is that an intake worker might discuss the intervention group with each homeless individual and offer him/her the choice of being in the group or not. Here the practice principle the worker would be following would be client self-determination. Under these circumstances if those in the intervention group did better, study findings might be confounded by the differences in client motivation between the two groups rather than the content of the psycho-ed program or the interaction of the program and the motivation that clients brought to it.

Each of the foregoing practitioner departures from random assignment illustrates what researchers call "threats to internal validity". What this means is that practitioner behaviors that might undermine our ability to justifiably claim that the intervention did what we hoped it would do. More specifically, internal validity is the extent to which you are certain that the intervention that you think explained the difference in the observed post-intervention behavior (the O in the diagram) did in fact make the difference.

Why are we telling you all this if RCTs and efforts to guard against threats to validity also threaten practice? Two reasons. First, by understanding each of these strategic options and the underlying reasons for them, you can pick and choose from among them and construct a PBR design that works for you and your purpose. Second, thinking about these research issues helps you reflect on what you do in practice and why. Hence, knowing what program and practice assumptions are implicit in yours and your co-workers' practice decisions is valuable in itself.

Alternatively, in order to make strategically mindful compromises of ideal research principles for PBR purposes, a practitioner should learn as much as possible from her/his own practice research efforts and s/he must consider and constructively work with all threats to validity that researchers hope to avoid.

Threats to internal validity

In their classic research text written a half-century ago, Campbell and Stanley (1963) were the first researchers to compile a list of all the major threats to internal validity. These were and still are:

- history
- instrumentation
- maturation
- selection
- experimental mortality

- statistical regression
- testing.

These "threats" exist in every research study and are not unique to PBR. However, the informed PBR practitioner needs to know about them and what they mean, even if only to have an effective and empowered dialogue with a research consultant or to thoroughly document the limitations of your study. As important, particularly when you are not working with a consultant, is that you take these threats into account when you are conducting and making inferences from your own PBR studies.

History

History is anything that happens during the course of your study that is not part of your intervention (the independent variable) that could affect the outcome (the dependent variable). For example, perhaps as a result of participating in the psycho-ed program individuals learn of another program where vocational training is available and begin participating in that program before the psycho-ed sessions are completed. Another possibility is that there is a fire in the housing units in which participants live or a key trainer becomes ill and is replaced. It is easy to see how these unanticipated occurrences could "contaminate" your study and impact participant behavior in positive or negative ways.

Instrumentation

Instrumentation is concerned with whether any of the testing instruments that you are using to measure your variables change in a systematic way during your study. An example of this would be if the indicators or measures or standards that you were routinely using to measure psychiatric symptomatology or treatment compliance or substance use were altered over the course of the study. So for example, if a new issue of the DSM were published wherein diagnostic criteria that were germane to the homeless mentally ill in your study were suddenly changed.

Maturation

Maturation refers to naturally occurring changes that happen to participants during the course of your study, this is especially relevant in longitudinal studies that take place over a long period of time and with participants that are at ages when considerable developmental changes occur, for example during early childhood or adolescence. So, for example, if some of the homeless, mentally ill individuals in your sample were older adults and becoming demented as a result of a combination of age, a history of addiction, and economic deprivation, these factors might have an independent effect on your outcome measures over a period of a year – particularly among the older clients.

Selection

Selection bias occurs when your experimental and control groups differ in some systematic way. We discussed this form of "bias" at length at the beginning of this section on threats to validity in the context of practice versus research integrity. However, we did not exhaust the many ways in which explanatory designs might be subverted.

So in the psycho-ed example, it is possible that chance occurrences might affect who is assigned to which group. Hence, based on the desire to start a psycho-ed group as soon as possible, program staff might sign up the first suitable home-less, mentally ill, substance-abusing clients who make themselves available for the housing program. The control group might then be made up of those requiring further outreach. By taking the first 20 people to arrive to make up the experimental group and the next 20 people to arrive as the comparison group, you may be building in other differences that might inadvertently influence outcome other than those directly associated with your intervention. Here again, it is easy to see how practice and program imperatives as well as wholly accidental factors might represent a "threat" to the "ideal" research design.

Experimental mortality

Experimental attrition (mortality) occurs when a particular type of participant, perhaps the very high functioning drop out of your study at a higher rate than others, or when the types of participants that drop out from the experimental group are different from the types of participants that drop out from the control group. Although attrition is common in all sorts of practice-research studies, it becomes a serious threat to the inferences one can make from study findings when the resulting differences between the two groups are associated with the outcomes in which we are interested. For example, the potential impact on outcome could be quite large if the people who drop out of the psycho-ed group are those who are most seriously disturbed or addicted or both. This could lead to the impression that psycho-ed is more effective than it truly is. Alternatively, if for some reason, the more troubled clients drop out of the control group, the incorrect conclusion that we might draw from our findings is that the intervention is less effective than it really is.

Researchers have a special way of designating these errors of inference. Type I error or "false positives" are errors that occur when you think an intervention is having an impact when it really isn't. Type II error, also known as "false negatives" are those when you infer that an intervention isn't having an impact when it truly is. Here again, differences between researchers and practitioners become evident since researchers tend to be more cautious and conservative about ascribing a benefit to an intervention than are practitioners who are understandably eager to find positive intervention outcomes. Despite these differences in perspective, knowing about what conclusions to properly draw from a set of PBR findings is important for every PBR practitioner.

Statistical regression

For researchers, regression ("statistical regression towards the mean") means something analogous but different from what it means to psycho-dynamically oriented clinicians. For clinicians it refers to a return to unwanted behaviors associated with an earlier stage of psychological development as when a traumatized child returns to bed-wetting. For researchers it refers to the natural tendency for very high or very low quantitative scores to move towards the middle over time. For example, no matter how smart a student is, it is highly unlikely that s/he will continually score 100% on every test s/he takes throughout college. At some point his/her score will regress (move closer) to the average.

To bring it closer to home, if you scored 100 percent on your first 20-item research quiz, it is quite likely that on the next one you might miss a question and score 95 percent. The same is true if you have an extremely low score on your first research quiz; chances are you will get more questions right on the next test even if you are totally guessing. So, in studies that initially involve outliers – extremely high or extremely low scores – subsequent test scores will move those participants towards the middle in repeated tests.

If, in our psycho-ed example, participants were given tests of their knowledge about pharmaceuticals and/or illegal drugs and their side-effects, and they scored extremely low at the beginning of the workshop, subsequent tests would suggest knowledge acquisition that might not be truly there. This tendency of scores to move towards the middle will thereby affect our ability to detect the true impact of an intervention.

Testing

Testing sounds like a routine part of every evaluation study. But when referred to as a "threat" it is about the impact that having been exposed to questions or a test once will have on your answers to the same question the next time you are asked it – even if you are not really learning anything or changing in any way. Thus, you may remember the answers that you gave the previous time you took the test. On a "multiple choice" test, for example, you may recall that last time you took the test, you frequently selected the option 4 as your answer and this time you may say "I'm a '4' so I'll pick that answer again". On the other hand, you may recall that you answered 4 but be motivated to show "improvement" or change, in this case you may purposefully select 5 as your answer in order to "show" that change without fully reading the questions and reflecting on the most appropriate answer at that moment. This tendency for our previous scores to influence our current scores is referred to as the "testing effect" threat to internal validity. In the psycho-ed example, in a Time-1/Time-2 study of risk behaviors, respondents who may want to please for good or not-so-good reasons, e.g. gratitude or manipulation, might positively misrepresent their risk-taking behaviors at Time 2 – perhaps because they are grateful and want to please or perhaps because they fear being dropped from the housing program if their behaviors don't improve.

Each of the foregoing threats to internal validity illustrates how they may distort what you see as the outcome of the study, masking the actual reality in some way. The goal with experimental and quasi-experimental designs is to reduce threats to internal validity as much as possible, so that you can be as sure as possible that any change that you observe in the dependent variable (the outcome you are measuring – Y) was really caused by your independent variable (your intervention or agent of change – X). When threats to internal validity do exist, which is often the case in PBR, it is important to either: anticipate them as much as possible in your study design; test for them statistically in your data analysis; or, at the very least, acknowledge the potential for them to exist and to try to account for them in the conclusions that you draw from your findings.

DESIGN FEASIBILITY

Practice imperatives

Perhaps the single most important consideration in choosing a PBR design is feasibility, i.e. how likely is it that the design will be implemented? As we have suggested earlier, the most important principle in selecting a PBR research design is to be sure to honor practice imperatives over research imperatives. That is, the research design selected should fit most comfortably with the existing practice model or should be easily adapted.

A second PBR principle here would be to choose the most "rigorous" design possible within the constraints of the practice setting and practice protocols. Unfortunately, as we have seen, the RCT "ideal" held up to practitioners by research academics and RBP advocates as the "gold standard" is rarely congruent with practice imperatives. Of the six values in the National Association of Social Workers Code of Ethics, service is listed first (NASW, 2008).

Another practice value and set of skills that practitioners feel is violated or dismissed by RCTs is differential assessment – i.e. matching the client, group, organization or community with the most suitable intervention (Epstein, 2010). Random assignment, which is essential to the RCT design, eliminates the practitioner's professional judgment about who should receive what treatment? Hence, as a practitioner-researcher you might object to the implementation of an RCT if the design requires that you use randomization to determine which clients receive which services, as opposed to utilizing your thoughtful clinical assessment. From a practitioner's view of our ethical code, the only context in which an RCT is appropriate is where the practitioner actually questions whether non-intervention is better than intervention and where there is concern that practitioner assessment is potentially worse than random assignment. For better or for worse, this set of beliefs rarely occurs among practitioners. After all, if you thought your assessment was not useful and your intervention wasn't helpful then you probably wouldn't be practicing.

On the other hand, the model for the use of RCTs comes from the testing of pharmaceuticals, in which the "placebo" control (sugar pill) is quite reasonably less damaging than an experimental drug. In order to further their case, RCT, RBP and

EBP advocates like to emphasize the limits, irrationality and potential for damage that practitioner judgment and "non-empirically supported" interventions can cause (Gambrill, 2010; Pignotti and Thyer, 2009). But as we have seen, RCTs are not the only way to empirically test and assess how effective social work interventions are.

Strategic compromises in study design

So, in our example of homeless, mentally ill individuals the study design calls for a pre- and post-test of relevant psycho-ed knowledge and risk behaviors, and is strengthened by the presence of a comparison group that receives housing services but no psycho-ed intervention. Of course, the effects of the intervention could be distorted if participants in the intervention group start sharing their information with those in the comparison group. Practitioners who understandably want all their clients to benefit as much as possible from program involvement might not consider that a "threat" though researchers clearly would.

Alternatively, employing a cross-over design, might be a solution satisfying everyone. In this design the individuals who were in the non-psycho-ed group at first would be put on a waiting list and offered a psycho-ed intervention immediately after the first group had completed theirs. in this way, every person in the program could benefit from psycho-ed and we would have even more evidence of whether it worked or not. In order to make this inference however, it would be imperative that both psycho-ed offerings were essentially the same.

Ultimately, however, the decision to have a comparison group and/or to employ a cross-over design might come down to very practical decisions about resources and costs, space availability and money for trainers, etc. Having more clients in the psycho-ed group to begin with would enlarge the potential pool of the pre- and post-test group, which offers its own advantages for statistical purposes. If, on the other hand, there was not time and space to run groups for all the homeless, mentally ill, substance abusing clients needing services at once and a naturally occurring wait list was available to serve as a comparison group, then that design would be selected as it could add an extra dimension of information to the study within the bounds of "practice as usual". With a comparison group we could consider not just changes in risk behavior before and after the group but also in comparison to the scores of similar homeless, mentally ill individuals who were not exposed to the group experience.

Time

A key factor in deciding a design is the time available or appropriate for the study, which will determine whether the study is longitudinal or cross-sectional. A longitudinal design is a study that collects data over time in an effort to capture the effects of an intervention process or program. So for example, we might assess risk and resiliency factors among homeless mentally ill residents in a shelter on a monthly basis in an effort to know the degree to which they are benefiting from the housing, counseling and placement services offered them. Obviously, this would be a time-consuming and labor-intensive design.

If we don't have the resources to conduct a longitudinal study, or if changes in the same individuals over time are not central to our research question, we might instead choose a cross-sectional design. The latter involves collecting data at one point in time from clients who have been in the program for different time periods – i.e. one month, two months, three months, etc. Comparisons of these different cohorts would be the basis for inferences about how the program impacts clients. This is a much more efficient, less costly and less potentially intrusive design than following clients on a monthly basis over the course of, say, a year in a shelter program. (Though it might have the additional clinical benefit of assuring that each client is seen and assessed by a worker at least once a month.)

The simplest kind of cross-sectional study does not make any attempt to explain what happened before or after anything, but simply reports the situation at that moment. So, if you want to determine who your agency is serving and you do a cross-sectional study you will describe your clients at this one point in time. Such a study makes no effort to tell you who your clients were a year ago, nor who they will be next year, nor how people change over time, but it does tell you who they are right now.

In a cross-sectional approach, resources permitting, every resident could be assessed in a single day. While this degree of efficiency is certainly appealing, it is important to remember that the evaluative inferences that one might draw from all the data collected and comparisons made would rest on the assumption that the program itself had remained stable over the course of the year and that there hadn't been significant attrition of residents over time.

Hence if our homeless mentally ill clients were medically compliant at the completion of the psycho-ed group, that finding would be highly relevant to practitioners. Whether it could be proven that it was the housing services or the psycho-ed group or some combination of the two that made the difference would be of lesser significance to the practitioner than to the researcher. Better still for everyone concerned if we re-assessed these clients at 6 and 12 months after the group thereby transforming the study into a longitudinal, outcome-only design. The data collected in this study could answer questions about what happened to the homeless, mentally ill clients' medication compliance (and risk and resiliency behaviors) over time.

In many cases, the first step for a PBR study is to study the problem in an after-only or a cross-sectional way and then build on, add to, or replicate the study using either the same or a slightly more rigorous PBR design. Whatever research you do and design you choose, you will learn more about your practice – your objectives, your interventions and the outcomes you are achieving. Considering these design issues and matching your selection to your study purpose will aid you in reflecting upon that practice long before you have collected any data.

Simply stated, in PBR the focus is on what will inform practice the most, while disrupting practice the least. But resources and the cost of conducting research are also important in choosing a design.

SUMMARY OF KEY CONCEPTS

In this chapter we have discussed various RBP and PBR design options and their strengths as well as their limitations. In this context, we introduced the concept of internal validity or your certainty that the outcome you are measuring (the dependent variable) is caused by the intervention you are testing (the independent variable). The seven major "threats" to internal validity were therefore described: history, maturation, testing, instrumentation, statistical regression, selection, and experimental mortality. The chapter also focused on feasibility factors that impact your PBR design selection, and practice imperatives. Most importantly, we have emphasized how selection of a PBR research design should be based on a guiding principle that involves seeking practice-based research knowledge in a manner that is least likely to compromise practice principles and service to clients and the community.

Chapter 5

The PBR literature review –
when and how to do it

Purpose

In RBP one always begins a research inquiry with a review of prior research literature. That's not the case with PBR. This chapter describes how review of the research literature fits into the PBR process and explains the logic behind deciding when you conduct the literature review. More specifically, this chapter discusses the difference between:

- conducting a literature review for informing your PBR study;

- conducting a literature review for choosing an evidence-based intervention;

- writing a literature review for publication purposes.

To make clearer how prior research can inform the PBR process, we explore some of the key features of each of these uses of prior research.

INTRODUCTION

Throughout this book we have described differences between PBR and other more "traditional" research models. In doing so, we have focused especially on the PBR imperative to honor practice protocols ahead of research protocols, and to employ strategic compromise in attempting to balance those imperatives when they come into conflict. This chapter focuses on some additional differences between PBR and other research models, namely a strategic approach to the purpose and placement of the literature review. Though in prior chapters, we have talked about "strategic compromise" in other aspects of PBR decision-making, in this chapter we will discuss the strategy behind deciding when to conduct the literature review in PBR, while definitely not compromising on the quality of that review.

In conventional research used in social work schools and models of evidence-based practice (EBP) proposed for practitioners, a systematic review of literature occurs very early in the process of problem formulation and/or intervention selection. Indeed, in EBP, the cornerstone of intervention selection is the systematic review of the research literature (Roberts and Yeager, 2004). In PBR, by contrast, the review of literature is usually not done until after the problem formulation process has been completed. At what point after the completion of the problem formulation depends somewhat on the purpose and methodology of your study, as we will discuss in a moment. The reason for this differential placement is that the key purpose of the literature review in PBR is different from that in other research-based processes. This chapter will detail this difference in purpose, and then set out to provide some guidance on how to conduct a PBR literature review, while bearing in mind the dynamic nature of PBR as well as the influence of information technology.

Within this chapter we will also discuss key components in writing a literature review, although we realize that as a practitioner-researcher you may have little interest in publishing your study findings in a peer-reviewed journal that routinely requires a discussion of prior research conducted on your topic. Should you wish to seek publication, however, it's important for you to know how. But that is only one of a number of ways to share your PBR experience and disseminate your research findings, which are discussed in Chapter 13.

PURPOSE OF THE LITERATURE REVIEW IN PBR

PBR studies evolve inductively out of practice decision-making needs rather than deductively from abstract theoretical interest. The latter approach is typical of academic research-based studies such as PhD dissertations. EBP literature reviews have a more pragmatic purpose, i.e. intervention selection, but assume that other than a critical and comprehensive literature review to inform practice, you the practitioner will not be conducting research of your own. Or if you do, it will only be to evaluate the impact of your intervention. This last expectation may be seen as a mid-point between an RBP model in which the practitioner is solely a consumer and applier of prior research and PBR in which the practitioner actively engages in research that may inform practice at any stage – from identifying client needs to assessing client outcomes.

In ideal conceptions of EBP (Gambrill and Gibbs, 2009), the EBP practitioner uses research knowledge and critical assessment of prior research to select interventions, and is an evaluator of the interventions ultimately used. In our experience, however, EBP practitioners do not take this final PBR step. Why they don't is a matter of speculation. It could be that dreaded "research reluctance" rearing its head again or it could be a matter of expectation by academic EBP advocates and EBP programs that place practitioners in the role of research consumers at best, or manualized practice implementers at worst. In the latter instance, the EBP practice manual is based on the program designer's prior research review and the practitioner is reduced to a "bureaucrat" with limited discretionary authority or opportunity for clinical creativity.

In PBR, practitioners are seen as capable of conducting their own research and of conducting a review of prior literature. However, this is not the starting point and is not required as a question-framing tool in the same way it is in other RBP models. Moreover, our focus is on generating new knowledge and applying existing knowledge specific to the practice setting in which the practice is being conducted. In that sense, PBR expects more of the practitioner but in so doing empowers practitioners as legitimate contributors to (not just consumers of) knowledge. However, while it is true that PBR study results have application to other settings, the main point of PBR is to solve an immediate practice problem. Therefore, our PBR problem emerges from the practice context (as we described in detail in Chapter 2), not from an identified gap in the literature as in academic research, or the search for a specific practice intervention as in EBP. Hence, a research literature review is not necessary in order to refine your research problem for your PBR study. Instead, you do that by examining your practice and deconstructing the very specific aspect of practice that you are trying to understand better.

It is important to note, however, that we are not saying you can't look at the literature before developing your practice-research problem. In fact, as a well-informed practitioner who reads professional journals and books you should already have a sense of the relevant literature and the state of the knowledge in your field of practice. What we are saying is that while such background information may be useful, it is not necessary to the shaping of the researchable problem from a PBR perspective. We also believe that in preparing you to be a practitioner-researcher you will be more likely to routinely and appreciatively read professional journals and research in the future. (We can but hope!)

We confess to a secondary reason for not including the literature review in the PBR process until after the practice problem has been sharpened or even until the study design is well formulated and under way. This is because conducting a comprehensive review of prior research can put you off! Often the prospect of sifting through the now dizzying amount of available research in lunch hours and after work can feel overwhelming and can serve as a barrier to practitioner-conducted research before it even starts. Theoretical discussions may seem endless and hopelessly abstract. Statistical analyses may seem impossible to ever comprehend. Moreover, online computer searches of the literature that are not informed by a clear idea of what you are looking for can generate an enormous output of vaguely related studies or nothing at all. More often than not, the former is overwhelming and the latter disappointing. Both are depressing and feed a sense of research hopelessness and incapacity.

In our collective experience of teaching PBR to social work students and providing PBR consultation to social work and allied health practitioners in all sorts of settings and in several countries, once the PBR process is well under way practitioner-researchers are more actively motivated to find out what literature might be helpful and have a more refined idea about how it might be helpful. Put simply, it's easier to find the energy to do the "lit search" once you have already "invested" in your own project with your own client or client population in mind.

CONDUCTING A LITERATURE REVIEW VERSUS WRITING A LITERATURE REVIEW

After all this discussion, and before we go any further, we have to address the "elephant-in-the-room" question "what exactly is a literature review?" In fact, the term "litera-ture review" can create confusion because it has two slightly different meanings. First, conducting a literature review or searching the literature, refers to the process of searching for books, articles, conference proceedings, other documentation and infor-mation to determine what knowledge exists that is relevant to your study topic. So, for example, if you are planning on studying which symptoms of post-traumatic stress disorder (PTSD) are most prevalent in your clients who are survivors of domestic violence, you would conduct a search for information related to that topic to give you a sense of what is known to date about the type and prevalence of PTSD symptoms in survivors of domestic violence (we will discuss exactly how to do that in a moment).

A second meaning of "literature review" is the written synthesis of all of the infor-mation that you gathered when you conducted your literature review, usually for pres-entation in a publishable research report. The goal of writing a literature review is to synthesize the relevant information that you gather about your topic, to present it in a way that creates a logical picture of what is known, and also identifies what is not known about your area of study to this point. A statistical approach to synthesizing the quantitative RCT research literature on a particular topic to show the ways in which the findings are consistent or different is called meta-analysis (Littell, Corcoran, and Pillai, 2008). The authors may even do a power analysis to show the strength of the findings. EBP texts detail specific instructions for how to use meta-analyses and other quantitative studies to conduct "systematic reviews" with the purpose of selecting practice interventions (Roberts and Yeager, 2004). To our thinking, "manuali-zation" of practice guidelines in which academic "experts" do the intervention selection "for" practitioners represents an unfortunate assumption that practitioners cannot be counted on to properly read research and/or don't have the capacity to understand it.

In the remainder of this chapter, we will explore the mechanics of both conducting a PBR literature review and writing one. The EBP approach is contained within the former and the academic is contained within the latter. Above all our hope is to be pragmatic and useful to you and to your clients.

STARTING THE LITERATURE REVIEW PROCESS

Whether you are simply thumbing through the latest issue of a recent social work journal or you are contemplating an online, computerized search of every journal imaginable, you have to have very clear answers to two questions:

- What is the topic that you want to search?
- Why are you doing it?

It follows that the more specific you are about your research question, the more able you will be to refine your search to the very specific theoretical concepts, methodological requirements, research findings and practice applications that are directly related to your PBR study.

More specifically, are you looking for epidemiological information about the existence of the problem you are interested in among certain populations? Are you looking for available assessment and/or evaluation research instruments to use directly and/or to develop your own instrument? Are you doing a more comprehensive search to understand what theoretical knowledge exists about the causes of the problem or theories about amelioration? Are you looking for sampling strategies and ways to engage participants in providing you with data? Are you looking for the latest research evidence about the effectiveness of various kinds of intervention approaches as in conventional EBP approaches? Are you looking for studies concerning those who do poorly with these "evidence-based" approaches – a question that EBP proponents rarely ask (Lo, *et al.*, in press).

Our main point here is that you use your understanding of your own PBR problem and study requirements to refine the terms that you use to search the databases, and you use your understanding of your purpose to help you to filter the information that emerges from your search. Moreover, you use that understanding in selectively reading and attending to those articles and books that you do read. Nothing is more time-consuming, discouraging and less possible than reading every word of every article that might possibly be related to your study. You don't read a menu that way in ordering a meal and you don't conduct a literature review that way either.

In general then, when conducting a literature review you may be trying to:

- identify variables in your area of study;
- gather theoretical and conceptual information about those variables;
- gather empirical data (research findings) about those variables;
- gather information about the types of research methods that have been used in similar studies while also assessing the strengths and weaknesses of those methods that have been used;
- identify instruments/measures/interview protocols that have been used – and also information about their strengths, weaknesses, validity and reliability.

SEARCHING DATABASES AND OTHER SOURCES OF INFORMATION

Traditionally, literature searches involved searching through book catalogues, journal contents pages, and perhaps newspaper catalogues to see what has been published on your area of study, or areas that were similar. However, with the explosion of technological advances and the accompanying onslaught of information, a literature search has become more of an information search. In fact, while we have constructed this section on conducting a literature search, we recognize that the rapid advancements in information technology mean that we can only give you an idea of how to search for relevant information. It may well be that some of the databases or techniques that we describe in this chapter will be replaced or modified by the time you read this book and are searching for literature related to your study – just as Yahoo! was replaced by Google as a favorite "search engine" and now Bing would like to replace Google. So we will give you basic suggestions and ideas about how to use these search devices, but you should check to see whether there have been advancements or changes in the way you should access information before you begin your actual search.

While for us old-timers, nothing can replace the joy of thumbing through recent issues of various journals in a periodical section of a library or the pleasure of wandering through the library "stacks" to look at "actual" rather than "virtual" books, pawing painstakingly through index cards and card catalogues in the libraries of our student days was always a drag. For you dear reader, the world is now your informational oyster. And it is available to you every month of the year and accessible from home in your jammies, on your iPod, BlackBerry, PC, Mac, iPad, Kindle and possibly coming soon on your wristwatch and in your soapdish.

Sophisticated search engines such as EBSCO, PsycInfo, MEDLINE, and Social Work Abstracts, can rapidly rifle through enormous quantities of journals and provide you with a comprehensive list of articles potentially relevant to the topic that you asked them to search. The key here is that the quality of your search depends on the combination of databases you use and the search terms you request. The two dangers in searches are that you will be so specific that you will identify only limited information, or you will be so broad that you will access far too much information. In fact, database searches have become so efficient that you can quite quickly become overwhelmed. Being overwhelmed is especially likely if you are studying very common broad terms like anxiety, depression, or substance abuse.

Given the potential to drown in reams of hard copy or less environmentally destructive but eyesight destroying online output, understanding how to use key words in your literature search is essential in both your and the planet's survival. Alternatively, a search that is too specific inevitably leads to an informational "black hole". To avoid each of these unfortunate and frightening possibilities, you need to master some "survival in cyberspace" techniques and know something about how all this information gets there in the first place.

When contemporary authors submit articles for publication, most journals routinely ask them to write a brief abstract and to list several key words that they can use to cross-reference the article for search purposes. So an article titled "Understanding the social work role in ethical decision-making in hospital settings" may have "ethical decision-making", "social work", and "health care" as its key words. If you were interested in ethical decision-making and you entered that as your search term, then this article would pop up in the list of results as one of your choices.

Databases vary in the types of articles that they access, some access education related materials, others focus on medicine, and others focus on social work. For most social work research it is good practice to search a range of different databases beyond social work since relevant information may be housed with sociology, psychology, medicine, education, or even business. Databases also vary in the way that they present material for you to review, some provide the title, the author(s), the journal that it was published in, and the publication date, while others also provide an abstract for you to review or even the full text of the article.

Here, it's important to remember that the author is a fallible human being (despite what may be an impressive trail of prior peer-reviewed publications) and that the key words chosen were not chosen with your study in mind. So relying on key words, and even the abstract alone, might lead to overlooking material that will be helpful to you. So, you need to quickly "screen" those articles that that look as though they might have relevant material, while maintaining an awareness of why you are looking at the article.

When sifting through the abstracts and articles that come up during your search, it is important to keep asking yourself about the relevance of the articles to the concepts in your study. If your search is turning up a high volume of articles that have only limited relevance to your study, then you need to add some more specific terminology to your search. Sometimes for example you may want to join two search terms together using "AND". For the search we mentioned earlier this may mean combining PTSD AND domestic violence. If you search just PTSD or just domestic violence then you may get a number of broad results, but if you combine the two you should retrieve only highly relevant references. You should of course include both post-traumatic stress disorder and PTSD in your search as some authors may write the term in full while others may use the acronym. Sometimes when you are searching, your topic is so specific that you yield either very few or even no results. If this is the case then you have to broaden your search topic(s) or even begin to search the next best thing – a similar topic that may at least have some relevant information.

So, if PTSD and domestic violence don't yield many results when combined then the broader term of "trauma" combined with domestic violence may yield more hits. The idea is that you would continue searching looking at the next most similar topic to see if there were relevant information or research methodology suggestions that may be informative for your study. If you find that an author or authors seem to have published a number of articles in your area of interest, then you can also conduct a search by author to see what you find. Another way to broaden your search can be to add an asterisk to the trunk of your search terms. When you add an asterisk to the stem of the work it indicates that you would like to search all variations of the term. So for example a search for ethic* would yield results for ethic, ethics, and ethical, while a search for depress* would yield references to depressed and depression.

Social work librarians are still an excellent resource when conducting a literature search. They tend to stay up-to-date on which databases are the most comprehensive and may even know which ones are most likely to yield results in your particular area. They are also experts in identifying search terms and search parameters that can capture relevant studies with a broad enough net to be comprehensive, but not so broad as to overwhelm you by capturing a lot of articles that aren't directly relevant.

A disclaimer

As we noted earlier, technology is evolving at such a rapid pace that even as we write this we have no idea whether the databases and techniques that we refer to will still be active and appropriate by the time you are reading it, or referring back to it as you construct your PBR study, so we offer suggestions here, but also recommend that you consult with a librarian or research consultant for advice as to the most current sources of information and the techniques that are most efficient to guide your search.

Another relatively "low-tech" way to start is to go the latest *Encyclopaedia of Social Work* (NASW, 2008) to see what is written generally on the topic and to identify some beginning possible sources. You can also go to Google Scholar (www.

googlescholar.com) to see what pops up before you begin a more systematic database search.

Sometimes, if you are lucky, your online search will yield a relatively recent "review article" or meta-analysis that systematically reviews recent research as well as more theoretical writing about the topic. An additional value of such a find is that it might include references to books on the topic. Hence, it is important to remember that online search engines often refer only to published articles but not to books. Finding a recent book on your topic (which may never show up on a computerized search) can be extraordinarily helpful.

Of course, looking for a book relegates you to the even more primitive "cave-dweller" strategy of spending time in the library stacks or the risks of thumbing through recent journals in the periodical room of your school library. That may sound neanderthal but – you never know – you might even enjoy it.

WHAT ARE YOU LOOKING FOR?

When you are conducting your literature search you are looking typically for two different kinds of relevant articles and/or books – conceptual and empirical. Conceptual materials are those that discuss your topic from a theoretical perspective. Perhaps they discuss different theoretical explanations for the phenomenon you are interested in studying, or they offer a new cutting edge explanation or theoretical link between cause and intervention approach or between intervention and outcome. In essence, the conceptual, theoretical articles and books explain why a problem might exist and offer insight as to what your research in the area might find. Often these materials can be used to develop hypotheses or predictions related to what we think you will find in your research study.

Empirical materials on the other hand are those articles and books that report the findings from research studies. These findings may be quantitative, qualitative or a mixture of the two, but they are based on some form of systematic observation and data collection. (Some mistakenly equate "empirical" with quantitative research, but as "methodological pluralists" the meaning we employ is verifiable through data and that includes all kinds of data.) Hence, by their very nature empirical articles include data of some kind and provide a description, analysis and interpretation of the data in some kind of report, article or book which may appear online or in hard copy.

Research studies can be useful to you for four reasons. First, they can show you how others have conceptualized the same or a similar issue. Second, they identify the instruments, measures, sampling or other strategies that others have used in their studies. Third, they can provide support or refutation of your findings. If findings differ, other differences such as demographic characteristics, differences in intervention "dosage" and/or quality, differences in program setting, cultural variations, etc. might suggest explanations for the differences found. Finally, they may suggest ways in which their findings have been "translated" or incorporated into practice. Remember PBR studies begin with practice questions and end with practice utilization. PBR is never about research for its own sake.

STRATEGIES FOR ORGANIZING INFORMATION

When conducting a literature search it is important that you develop a strategy for organizing the information you find. You want to be able to locate articles that are relevant, based on topic or methodology. You also want to make sure that you have the full citation for the article, so that you can quickly and easily establish a reference list to accompany your work. If you proceed hastily at first not getting full information or developing a strategy to file and save your search results, you can waste a lot of time later as you try to recreate your searches and locate reference information. As our late colleague Roselle Kurland would frequently say, "when it comes to the literature review – make haste slowly".

Although we recommend a strategic approach to the timing of the literature review and to its uses, this is one place in which we do not recommend a "strategic compromise". Most importantly, this does not imply limiting the search to those articles which support your expectations and/or findings. The principle to observe here is the same principle that applies in RBP literature reviews, that is the review should be exhaustive and unbiased. In fact, you stand to learn more from reading those publications and findings that disagree with your own. They provoke you to think and reflect rather than rest on what you think you know.

You may wish to make two electronic copies of the articles that you find to be relevant, one to file by author and the other by topic (just be sure to capture the full citation including page numbers). You will also need to develop a strategy for organizing information that is available via a website or in a different format. It may make sense to write a list of relevant websites with a summary of their content. For citation purposes you will not only need a record of the content on the website that you wish to reference, but you will also need a record of the web address and the date that you accessed the site (this is because many sites are changing frequently and you are asserting that on the day you accessed the site this is what you found). One useful strategy is to generate a record of your visit by cutting and pasting the url or web address into a Word file, along with a record of the relevant contents of the site and the date that the information was retrieved.

TIMING THE LITERATURE REVIEW

In addition to already having a sense of the literature as an informed practitioner, you may also wish to consult the literature at other points as you develop your PBR study. For example, you may consult prior studies on yours or a similar topic to see what types of data-collection strategies have been used. Are previous studies qualitative or quantitative? Do they use instruments that might be useful for your study? Or, are there questions that could be adapted to work well in your case? Searching the literature to inform your data-collection method selection and instrument development is a much more targeted effort than a full systematic literature review.

By contrast, a more comprehensive literature search may be conducted after your methodological choices have all been made and your methodology has been fully established. When conducted at this point in the PBR process, the purpose may be to ensure that there are no significant omissions from your study's conceptualization, design, or instruments. You may also conduct a literature review after data collection is under way. A literature review conducted at this point in the process may be being used to guide data analysis to see what variable combinations, statistical procedures, or qualitative data-analysis strategies have been used. It may also be used at this point to inform the interpretation of the data. As you can see in PBR the timing of the literature review relates to a strategic decision about the point at which the literature will provide the most support for your study process.

Certainly, if you wish to publish your study as well as to use it within your agency practice, full and comprehensive literature reviews will be necessary. This places your study in the context of other comparable studies and maximizes the contribution it can make to the profession. Otherwise, we are talking about an agency report which narrowly focuses on your study findings and their local application.

WRITING A LITERATURE REVIEW

As we indicated earlier, doing a literature search for a PBR study, or doing a systematic review of the literature for an EBP intervention and writing a literature review are not the same thing. Writing a literature review may or may not be part of your PBR process. Usually a literature review is constructed for a professional publication or a grant application. So, for example, all of the published papers by practitioners who have conducted clinical data mining (CDM) studies have included written literature review sections (see, for example, Joubert and Epstein, 2005; Peake, Epstein and Medeiros, 2005; Blumenfield and Epstein, 2001). Likewise, published CDM studies that were grant-funded by the Soros Foundation and the National Kidney Foundation, required literature reviews for their grant proposals as well as for their peer-reviewed journal publications, (see, Dobrof *et al.*, 2006; and Dobrof *et al.*, 2001, respectively). However, if you don't choose to disseminate your findings via formal publication and are not pursuing funding in the same or a similar area, then you probably won't need to write a literature review. As we have already mentioned the purpose of writing a literature review is to provide a narrative synthesis of the relevant literature that is available about your area of interest. So when writing a literature review your responsibility to your audience is to identify the theoretical literature that has been written on your topic as well as empirical studies that have generated findings relevant to your study. In addition, you should identify similarities or consistencies that you find in the literature, while highlighting inconsistencies or contradictions either in the conceptual understanding or the research findings. In your literature review you should also identify existing gaps in the knowledge base, perhaps providing a rationale for your study and pointing towards the construction of your research questions.

STRUCTURING THE LITERATURE REVIEW – ANOTHER USE OF THE FUNNEL

Funnels can be very useful in the kitchen but they also have a place in PBR. In fact, most written literature reviews take the shape of a funnel, in that they start with very broad ideas related to the nature of the problem that is being studied and then get progressively narrower and more specific as the theoretical foundations of the study are identified, the empirical findings of other research studies are described and the gaps or open questions in existing knowledge are articulated. In RBP studies the funnel often ends with a hypothesis or set of hypotheses to be tested. More typically, in PBR studies the funnel ends with unanswered, practice-relevant questions.

Figure 5.1 offers a summary of the key points from both the theoretical and empirical literature, followed by a statement of the gaps in the literature for which we don't yet have the evidence. Finally, the summary finishes with your very specific research questions and, when appropriate, hypotheses that are being tested in your PBR study.

When describing the nature of your PBR problem, your goal should be to establish the importance of your topic, letting your readers know why they should care about the issue and therefore about your study. A good way to establish the importance of your problem is to use data to assert the prevalence of the problem. Providing some description of the population that is affected by the problem can also be useful to orient your readers to the scope of your problem.

Once you have established the problem and its importance, you should present definitions of any key concepts for your study so that your readers are clear about the way you are interpreting terms and using them within your literature review. Such definitions of key concepts are the nominal definitions that we referred to in Chapter 2. Having established the definitions for your study, you can refer back to them as you review the literature alerting your readers as to whether the studies you talk about are using similar or different definitions of those terms. The danger if we don't establish definitions is a tendency to make assumptions that we know what you mean and that the reader knows what we mean as well, when in fact we have different notions of the same concept. If you are looking at the impact of stress on family coping, then it would be easy for your readers to make assumptions about what you mean by "stress", "coping", and "family", but in fact each of these terms has numerous different ways of being defined.

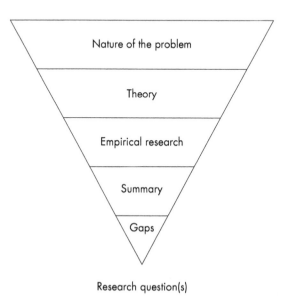

Research question(s)

FIGURE 5.1   The structure of the literature review

This point cannot be overemphasized because the same words can mean very different things in different types of enquiries. For example, to a psychoanalytically oriented social work clinician "rationalization" means something very different and perhaps diametrically opposed to what it means to a social work administrator or program planner grounded in organizational theory. In using that term, the former emphasizes the appearance of rationality applied to the irrational. The latter refers to a process by which organizational processes or program interventions are rendered more rational. Though their usages are opposed, in some sense, both are correct. Hence a reader would need to know what the term is intended to convey by the author. Clearly establishing your key definitions up front makes sure that there is no misinterpretation of your points.

In your literature review, once you have presented your PBR problem then you should discuss your understanding of the theoretical foundation of the concepts in your study and the potential relationships between them. That sounds quite fancy, but it follows very logically from your definitions. Having established your definitions, your theoretical section provides your justification for interpreting your concepts in that particular way. So, among the numerous theoretical interpretations of the concept of stress how do you understand it, and how does that relate to coping and the families that you are working with?

The key here is to be logical and theoretically consistent, so if you established a behavioural interpretation of stress, then you would look at behavioural treatments for stress and behavioural indicators of coping. On the other hand, a psychodynamic interpretation of stress factors would lead to a discussion of psychodynamic treatment interventions, and a psychodynamic understanding of coping. The theoretical section of your literature review orients the reader to your thinking around how the concepts in the study relate to each other, which helps to establish what relationships you expect to find in your study. The next step is to describe the research of others so that your readers understand what is already known about your topic, which also helps to establish what you might expect to find in your study.

Similar to the theoretical section, the empirical section of the literature review synthesizes the findings of studies available in your area of study. You identify the ways in which these other studies have been conceptualized, their methodology and their findings. However, in addition to synthesis you have an additional obligation when reviewing the empirical literature, which is evaluation.

Like the words "coping" and "rationalization", the term "evaluation" has different meanings. In this context, we mean evaluation of research rather than evaluation research. The former looks critically at published research, the latter at program implementation and outcomes, And not to put too fine a point on it, the word "critically" has different meanings. In RBP, it means finding all the flaws in a piece of research by comparing it against a "gold standard" ideal. This view is common to what some have referred to as "critical thinking" (Gambrill and Gibbs, 2009; Rubin and Parish, 2007). In PBR, however, "critically" assessing prior research means recognizing strengths as well as limitations of various forms of research. From the standpoint of research pedagogy, the negative approach is fostered by commonly-used research assignments in which students are asked to identify the "flaws" in studies. Accordingly, faculty might provide a study and ask students to identify 20 weaknesses in what the authors have done.

It's always easy to find flaws in someone else's research. As social work researchers working in real-world settings rather than in hermetically-sealed laboratories, none of us has ever done the "perfect study". And none of us ever will.

A more "strength-based" PBR approach to literature review involves appreciating the strengths as well as the limitations in prior research. With this more "appreciative" approach in mind, you should evaluate prior research by assessing the appropriateness of the methodology for your PBR question, the utility and fit of instruments or interview questions used to your purpose, the similarity or differences in the population from which the data was gathered and the population in your study, program and intervention differences, procedures for data analysis that were used and whether you have the resources and capacity to employ them yourself or with a research consultant, and the logic of the author's interpretation of the findings, and ultimately, their practice and program implications.

So, not only do you have to assess the appropriateness of the methods used in these other studies, but you also have to evaluate their applicability to your study. What is the "goodness of fit" between each study you review and the PBR study you intend to do? The good news is that as you read through the rest of this book you will become more fluent in the language of research, and therefore more equipped to assess the studies that your literature search uncovers. Box 5.1 provides a quick guide of things to look for as you are reviewing empirical literature. As we noted before, taking comprehensive notes and citation information the first time definitely pays off in the end. Box 5.1 is intended as a guide to help you to gather all the information you need to include a study in your review of literature.

When incorporating research studies into your literature review, the six factors identified in Box 5.1 should be reported for each study. In this way your readers can make their own assessment of the strength or weakness of the claims made by the author(s) of the study and its relevance to your study as well. The information from the six points might be synthesized down to one or two sentences or expanded to give a full description. In general, the more closely the research matches your PBR study the more fully you would want to describe each of the six features identified.

One final word of caution: when writing a literature review you should progress logically from idea to idea, integrating the information available on that idea before moving on to the next. You should not progress from author to author or study to study. When you do this then the reader has to try to make the connections between the studies and in turn link those ideas back to your study, which is precisely your job writing the literature review!

BOX 5.1   ASSESSING EMPIRICAL STUDIES: WHAT TO LOOK FOR IN OTHER RESEARCH STUDIES

Key factors to understand and report for each empirical/research study:

1 The research question
   a What was the main purpose of the study?
   b Were there any sub-questions?
   c What is the theoretical orientation of the study?

2 Sample
   a Who was the focus of the study?
   b Who was the sample and how representative was it of the population under study?
   c What was the gender, racial, ethnic, and age breakdown of the sample – how does that compare to the sample that you anticipate?

3 Design
   a What research design was used?
   b Was it quantitative, qualitative or mixed method?
   c Did it follow logically from the study purpose?

4 Measures/instruments/interview schedules used
   a Did the questions used conceptually match the variables being studied?
   b Were reliability and validity adequately established for any instruments used?
   c Were the instruments and questions used appropriate for the developmental and cultural background of the study sample?

5 Findings
   a Are the results reported substantiated by the data analysis reported?
   b What were the major findings of the study?

6 Application
   a What are the practice and program implications of the study findings?

SUMMARY OF KEY CONCEPTS

In this chapter we discussed the differential value of the search of the literature and the literature review. Each might occur at different points in the PBR process. We also discussed how to match the literature review purpose with its placement in the PBR process. We distinguished between conducting a review of the literature and writing a literature review. We note that in many cases you may not write a literature review as part of your PBR study. We described search engines, key-word searches, and ways to organize material when conducting a literature search, while cautioning that ways to access information are changing so rapidly that consulting a social work librarian can be invaluable. Next, we introduced one way to organize material for a written literature review and described key information that should be included when reporting on prior research studies. The subsequent chapters will discuss many of the research concepts that you will need to understand in order to evaluate the quality of the research that you discover during your literature search.

One final, final word of caution. Though we contend that conducting a PBR study does not require writing a review of the literature, if your research instructor requires it, just do it! You'll get nowhere justifying not doing it by quoting Dodd and Epstein. And very likely, you'll learn more about what you know and what you don't by doing it.

Chapter 6

Understanding basic differences in data-collection methods

Purpose

PBR is not just a theoretical stance about integrating practice and research. It's also a way of doing empirical research. By that, we mean gathering evidence of one kind or another and basing practice decisions on data. This chapter explores the different data-collection methods available to you for your PBR study, and some of the factors to consider in choosing a method that is right for your purposes

---

INTRODUCTION

This chapter introduces two different methods of data collection, both useful to you in conducting PBR studies. Qualitative data collection involves data collected and analyzed in words, while quantitative data collection involves data collected in numeric form and analyzed statistically. Both have their uses and they can be meaningfully combined in mixed-method PBR studies.

In doing PBR, it is essential that you develop the skills and flexibility to employ either or both quantitative and qualitative data-collection strategies when addressing your study questions. Ultimately, we're hoping that you won't think of yourself as either a "quantitative practitioner-researcher" or a "qualitative practitioner-researcher" but as a practitioner-researcher with a repertoire of both sets of research skills that can be applied creatively and appropriately to the practice-based questions you seek to answer. And yet with each method, as well as in mixed-method studies, questions of validity and reliability of the data need to be carefully considered.

Once you have determined your PBR question(s), the study purpose, and your study design, your next task is to identify the type of data that you want to gather, its source, and the tools that you are going to use to gather it. (Data is what we call the unprocessed and unrefined information that you will use to answer your practice-based questions.)

Data may be either quantitative or qualitative. If quantitative, it either comes in the form of numbers originally or is converted into numbers from some type of qualitative data, such as words, observations, etc. A person's age, for example or how many siblings they have, or how many counseling sessions they attend, or how soon their children are reunited with them from foster care, are all straightforward examples of numeric quantitative data. Alternatively, qualitative non-numeric data – such as whether a client or group of clients have achieved their treatment goals or what types of interventions they have received or their ethnic identification – can be converted into numerical data by assigning numbers to the different possible response categories.

Although no one has thought of a way to convert quantitative data into qualitative, when we have many quantitative client "data-points" over time, we can sometimes approximate a qualitative process of change with quantitative data. If we think about the way motion pictures or computer "streaming" are made up of multiple still images, this offers an analogy. A third alternative is that qualitative data in the form of words, metaphors, video images and direct observations may remain qualitative and be analyzed as such. For example, social workers' case notes, clients' verbal responses to interview questions, or observations of children's responses to play therapy are all examples of qualitative data that may be analyzed entirely qualitatively.

Another important distinction involves original or available data collection. Sometimes we have no alternative but to collect original data because existing data do not address the questions we are interested in studying. At other times, routinely available data can inform practice decision-making. Epstein (2010) has referred to the process of gathering and analyzing existing information as clinical data mining (CDM). In RBP preference tends to be given to original data collection. In PBR, since we are concerned about not intruding on practice or burdening clients while conducting research, preference is given to studies based on available data. Here again, the practitioner-researcher's repertoire should include both available and original data-gathering skills. Back to our original distinction, some PBR questions lend themselves more readily to quantitative data-gathering strategies, while others lend themselves more to qualitative strategies. Very often in PBR we find that the most comprehensive way to gather data about our question is to use both strategies, which we refer to as using mixed methods. Hence the idea that PBR is "methodologically pluralist" has been expanded beyond our original discussion to embrace quantitative, qualitative and mixed-method studies that involve original and available data collection. These various options are identified in Table 6.1.

DIFFERENT DATA-COLLECTION METHODS

An emphasis on gathering original quantitative data emerged from a positivist approach to research, the foundations of which are consistent with the notions of RBP (Epstein, 2001). Positivists believe in the objectivity of research. Hence, their understanding of epistemology is that it is possible to separate the knower from what can be

TABLE 6.1 Types of data collection

Data type	Data source	
	Available data	Original data
Quantitative		
Qualitative		
Mixed method		

known, which means that a study can be value-free. Ideally, if reality can be objectively observed then values are not involved or can be excluded. The positivist approach is a strong proponent of quantitative methods in social work research.

Post-positivists acknowledge that research can never be totally value-free, but attempt to minimize the intrusion of their own values by developing and using standardized quantitative instruments. Standardized research instruments provide statistical standards or norms against which it is thought possible to compare individuals of every social class, culture, ethnic group, etc. The IQ test and associated scoring is a classic example of such an instrument. While positivist beliefs have evolved through time, the central notion of post-positivists is still the idea that there are universal truths that can be uncovered and revealed through quantitative research – for example, which individual or group is more intelligent than which other individual or group.

EBP advocates strongly endorse post-positivist assumptions that it is possible for both researchers and practitioners to make generalizations about the effectiveness of social work interventions by critically reviewing research studies (McNeill, 2006; McNeece and Thyer, 2004; Mullen, 2004). Similarly, EBP proponents believe that researchers can make more rigorous research-based generalizations by statistically summarizing the results of multiple studies of practice that employ the same interventions and quantitative measures of treatment outcomes, preferably in the form of RCTs. They refer to this process of aggregating and summarizing the findings of multiple studies as meta-analysis (Littell, Corcoran and Pillai, 2008).

Practice-based researchers are much less concerned with coming up with findings that are generalizable to all practice settings and client populations than they are concerned about making decisions and inferences about their own practice-setting and client population. In this regard, we earlier commented that PBR comes closer to what Scriven (1995) has called formative evaluation rather than summative evaluation. Elsewhere, some have argued PBR in general and CDM in particular are less global and more local in their knowledge-generating aspirations (Chan *et al.*, 2009; Epstein *et al.*, unpublished manuscript under review).

Whether globally or locally applied, some concepts involve naturally occurring numbers, as in our previous examples of age, number of siblings, years of education and number of treatment sessions, whereas others do not. In instances where either the available or the original data are initially qualitative, an analytic approach to using these data might be to develop numerical scales that can be used to quantify (attribute a number to) them. Thus, we could count the number of problems clients identify at intake or the number of treatment goals they have attained upon treatment termination.

Some phenomena are more directly observable than others. It's one thing to infer that a client is depressed or anxious or has low self-esteem by observable but non-verbal behaviors but another thing to ask the client to self-report about less observable states. As a result, researchers have developed quantitative self-report scales to measure these inner states, attitudes and behaviors that might not lend themselves to direct observation. These might include sexual orientation, self-esteem, satisfaction with services and/or behaviors.

Some standardized quantitative scales are quite long and burdensome to complete. Others, called rapid assessment instruments (RAIs) are designed to be used in practice and require much less time and effort for a client to complete. There are a variety of quantitative data sources that can be used for PBR studies, many of which will be explored in Chapter 8. Quantitative sources include the standardized scales we just discussed, original surveys or questionnaires that are developed specifically for your research purposes, and routinely available quantitative data that are gathered as part of standard client intake, assessment, or evaluation forms.

On the other hand, qualitative data-collection methods are focused not on numbers but on words, actions and/or non-verbal cues. Qualitative data collection is consistent with a social constructivist approach to research and the notion that rather than just one truth there are, in fact, many truths which we each construct differently based on our interactions (Guba and Lincoln, 2008; 1994; 1989; Guba, 1990). Constructivist scholars and especially feminist researchers have contributed greatly to the developed thinking about the social construction of concepts and have refined the sophistication of qualitative methodology (see for example, Hill-Collins, 1990). Rather than reduce complicated concepts down to a single number or numerical score, qualitative research produces "thick descriptions" of how people experience their psycho-social problems, interventions and outcomes.

As with quantitative data, there are a variety of sources of qualitative data open to the practitioner-researcher, which will be explored in the next chapter. These include for example, in-person, telephone, video-conference, or instant messaging interviews; in-person or videotaped observations; and, existing documentation including case records, process recordings, and meeting minutes.

The practice example in Box 6.1 illustrates the way in which qualitative and quantitative PBR studies of depression might vary. The following section considers some of the strengths and weaknesses of qualitative and quantitative data-collection methods, so that you have a sense of the factors to consider when you are choosing one strategy or the other for your PBR study.

By contrast, a quantitative study of depression would employ a standardized quantitative instrument to measure depression such as the Beck Depression Inventory (Beck *et al.*, 1996), or Zung (1965) self-rated depression scale, the Hamilton (1980) Rating Scale for Depression, or the Geriatric Depression Scale (Yesavage *et al.*, 1983). As a practitioner-researcher, you would ask every client to complete the test every three months to see whether their depression scores had changed and in which direction. In both instances the goal of the study is to determine whether your or your program's intervention was successful in reducing symptoms of depression, but the methods used, and the type of data gathered to "measure" depression are very different. And while the logical structure of both studies is the same, analysis of the data would be quite different as well. Thus, the qualitative study would be based on client narratives whereas the quantitative study would be based on client numerical scores.

BOX 6.1   PRACTICE EXAMPLE

In a qualitative study evaluating an agency-based treatment approach for depression as a practitioner-researcher, you might conduct an intake interview with a client Sylvia who has become homeless to see how she describes her emotional status and whether her description matches common symptoms of depression. Then, after three months of psychotherapy, or participation in a job-training program or receiving help with finding housing or all of the above, you may conduct a repeat interview to see if there is any change in the way Sylvia describes her emotional state. You would repeat this process for all of the participants in the study, and you would analyze the assessments to see whether there were themes and patterns that emerged in either a positive or negative direction for depressive symptoms. You may even ask clients directly whether they feel depressed, and whether they think that treatment has helped them, and if so in what ways.

A mixed-method study approach might combine a single standardized instrument to quantify depression levels before, during and after treatment with the addition of qualitative interview data exploring how clients are feeling at each measurement point, and why.

COMPARING STRENGTHS AND WEAKNESSES OF QUANTITATIVE AND QUALITATIVE METHODS

In comparing qualitative and quantitative strategies of data-collection methods, it becomes apparent that a strength of one is often a weakness of the other. So we will discuss the advantages and liabilities of each in contrast with the other.

We will start by looking at one of the strengths of quantitative data methods, their efficiency in data collection, analysis and interpretation. In other words, with quantitative data you can reduce a lot of information quickly and communicate the results efficiently. For example, if you want to know whether or not clients in your agency's community support a local playground initiative, you can poll a large number of them with a self-administered quantitative questionnaire and then reduce the responses to a simple percentage breakdown for or against the initiative. So, perhaps you and other community-center co-workers distribute 3,000 self-addressed questionnaires under the doors of community residents asking if they support an initiative for the development of a playground in a particular location. If 1,000 respond and you find that 750 support the playground and 250 do not, you have reduced the opinions of 1000 people down to two numbers – 75 percent in support and 25 percent opposed. Knowing as well that only about 33 percent of those households surveyed responded helps determine how much credibility to give to the results. Unfortunately, there may be no way to know anything about the nearly 67 percent who did not respond but it's better than just assuming support because you and your colleagues thought that the community "needed" a playground.

However, while the ability to reduce a large amount of information is a strength of quantitative research, the drawback in this case is that you still don't have a sense of why people supported or opposed the initiative, or the degree to which they supported or opposed the project. Were the residents fervently in favor of the project or just on the positive side of indifference? And what explained their response to the initiative?

So, if instead of putting surveys under people's doors you conduct 50 qualitative telephone interviews about the playground initiative with households drawn from a local telephone directory, you may get a greater sense of the factors that influence the extent to which people support or oppose the initiative. You would determine which parts of the project people strongly support or oppose and most importantly why?

True, you would only know the opinion of 50 members of the community, and you wouldn't know how representative the opinions of your small sample of respondents are in relation to everyone else. (Sampling is one way we try to address that issue, as we will discuss in Chapter 9.) The capacity to provide rich and full description of community responses to the proposed project, as opposed to reducing concepts to a few numbers or percentages, is an oft-cited strength of qualitative techniques (Denzin and Lincoln, 2008; Padgett, 1998; Tutty, Rothery and Grinnell, 1996). However, the generalizations you can make about the degree of support from information gathered via relatively few qualitative interviews constitutes the primary weakness of this strategy. And yet, the information that you do have is so much richer and more "nuanced" in the qualitative than in the quantitative study.

A further example of the potential for qualitative data to capture more nuanced information can be considered utilizing an anxiety study of a single client. You may know from a quantitative assessment instrument that your client completed at intake and upon completion of treatment that her or his score on an anxiety scale has decreased during treatment. You may also know which particular questions on the anxiety scale seem to indicate improvements, and/or any that indicate worsening symptoms or dimensions on which there has been no change at all.

However, in talking to your client in a termination interview you may learn that her/his self-perception was that the level of anxiety actually increased during the first few weeks of treatment, but then began to subside and leveled off during the last few weeks and now was slighter higher than it had been. When asked why, the client might have had much to say about the building of trust, the ways in which treatment had been helpful once a "connection" was made and that now the client is somewhat anxious about going it alone.

Without overburdening clients with repeated administrations of the anxiety scale, you would completely lose the details of these more subtle shifts in symptoms and the reasons why with only the quantitative analysis. This ability to provide a deeper understanding of the treatment experience relative to the questions posed, and perhaps to account for some explanatory factors from each client or set of clients, is a definite strength of qualitative data collection.

Admittedly, a drawback of qualitative PBR strategies is that they tend to be very time- and labor-intensive for both clients and practitioner-researchers, precluding work with large samples. Given this, qualitative studies are often based on the experiences of relatively few people who are ideally, strategically selected to tell their own "stories". Consequently, we don't know the extent to which the experiences of clients to whom the study has given "voice" mirror the experiences of other clients. So, from the standpoint of generalizability (a concept we will discuss in greater detail in our chapter on sampling strategies) qualitative research has distinct disadvantages as compared with quantitative research.

In addition, advocates of quantitative research contend that in qualitative research there is no way to test the reliability of your data, their analysis and the inferences that you draw from them. Reliability refers to the extent to which measures are applied consistently and thereby produce consistent results. In Chapter 8, we shall see that there are statistical tests to measure the reliability of numerical scales but no such tests exist for qualitative analysis.

Using our client anxiety example, quantitative researchers would argue that reliability tests give us some confidence that people with similar quantitative anxiety scores actually experience comparable levels of anxiety and that people with very different anxiety scores have very different levels of anxiety.

Another advantage of quantitative data is that it allows for the application of both simple and sophisticated statistical analyses. Basic statistics can describe the percentage breakdown of variables as with our community playground polling example, as well as tell us which was the most common response and how varied responses were. Such statistics are often used to provide a description of an agency's clients based on available intake data (Peake, Epstein and Medeiros, 2005). In this way you would have a sense of the numbers and proportions of clients served based on age, gender, ethnicity, geographic location, socio-economic status, presenting problem, etc. More advanced statistics can be used to illustrate the nature and strength of relationships between variables, they can even "model" relationships statistically, and may be used to test predictions (see, basic and inferential statistics in Chapter 12). A major advantage of these statistical techniques is that they can show time-trends in the data and can explore, test and draw data-driven conclusions about complex relationships and communicate them in relatively simple, numerical ways.

And yet this strength is also a limitation. Ironically, proponents of qualitative research claim that "highly sophisticated" statistical analyses reduce complex issues and relationships to simplistic numerical expressions that don't capture the nuances of the individual's experiences and/or their reasons for answering questions in particular ways. Simple is good when reality warrants it. Simplistic is bad when it distorts and over-simplifies important practice information.

It is pointless to ask whether qualitative or quantitative research is better. The real question is better for what and under what conditions? Here again the concept "strategic compromise" is essential to PBR decision-making. As a practice-based researcher you must understand the purpose of your study, and weigh the extent to which your problem is most suited to qualitative analysis, as is often the case with exploratory and some descriptive studies, or whether you want to explore cause-and-effect relationships and need to rely on statistical analysis and quantitative methods. Do you want to generate a descriptive picture of the dimensions you ask about on your client intake form that can be translated into numeric items, and so choose a quantitative strategy or do you want to gather a more nuanced understanding of your client's experiences with your agency or even its intake process?

Often, students are drawn to one method of data collection or the other based on their personal styles of thinking and learning. In our experience as teachers, students with a science background tend to be "linear" thinkers and prefer quantitative studies. Those with humanities backgrounds tend to prefer qualitative studies. In fact, historically, there have been very strong sentiments expressed between the supporters of more post-positivist quantitative data collection (Gambrill, 1995; Berlin, 1990; Hudson, 1982) and those of more social constructionist or heuristic qualitative data-collection methods (Heineman-Pieper, 1986; 1986; Heineman, 1981), so much so that while the controversy was known academically as a heated debate (Peile, 1988), it was colloquially referred to as the paradigm "wars".

For the most part, social work researchers like ourselves have moved beyond these wars and have become appreciative of the particular advantages as well as the disadvantages of each method. And, while some maintain a strong allegiance to one or another strategy, many including us have come to recognize the value of each, utilizing quantitative, qualitative or a combination of data-collection strategies as seems most appropriate for the PBR problem at hand. For that reason, we encourage you to push yourself to become familiar with and practice both sets of strategies so that you can let the PBR problem rather than your comfort level dictate your choice of data-collection strategy.

SUMMARY OF KEY CONCEPTS

This chapter introduced the distinction between qualitative data, which occurs and remains in non-numeric form such as words and images, and quantitative data, which occurs naturally or is converted into numeric form. The potential advantages and disadvantages of both types of data were explored along with the idea that a strength of quantitative data was a limitation of qualitative data and vice versa. This chapter also discussed the ways in which one or the other type of data collection, or a combination of both may be appropriate for your PBR study.

Now that we have considered the strengths and limitations of the two major types of data (i.e. qualitative and quantitative) that can be gathered, and their philosophical origins, the following two chapters will explore specific data-gathering techniques for each type of data. For reasons that do not imply preference, we begin with qualitative and then move on to quantitative and mixed-method approaches.

Chapter 7

Qualitative data gathering

Purpose

Qualitative data takes the form of words, metaphors or observed behaviors. This chapter explores the three useful PBR strategies for gathering qualitative data – interviews, observations, and content analysis. The chapter also explores key data-gathering concepts (e.g. reliability and validity) and applies them to qualitative data collection.

INTRODUCTION

There are different ways to generate or access qualitative data for PBR studies. Although RBP studies emphasize quantitative data collection, many sociologists, anthropologists and other social scientists routinely conduct qualitative research. What sets qualitative PBR studies apart from both RBP and social science approaches is that qualitative PBR allows your practice and programming to continue without major adjustments for research purposes.

For example, while knowledge of qualitative data-gathering principles might help you to improve the reliability and consistency of your clinical interviews, in order to generate more researchable qualitative data, it would not entail asking questions that are not clinically relevant. Thus minor enhancements in interviewing or coding protocols should not interfere with or compromise your practice priorities. If anything, it will improve your practice because it will add to your reflectiveness and consistency as a practitioner. Alternatively, you may choose a qualitative CDM strategy to "mine" available qualitative data from case records for PBR study purposes (Epstein, 2010). By conducting content analysis of records of practice that has already taken place, research requires no intrusion on your practice and adds no additional burden to your clients.

So, whether working qualitatively, quantitatively or mixing the two, the primary concern for PBR data collection remains being able to conduct practice-relevant research without disrupting practice. Given that some forms of conventional qualitative data gathering that we will discuss can be somewhat burdensome to your client-participants, then qualitative studies utilizing routinely conducted individual, family and group interviews, more systematic observation and "mining" available qualitative data from case records and other documents often fit well with PBR.

When selecting a qualitative data-collection strategy for your PBR study, you have to take into consideration several factors that we will also discuss in relation to quantitative data-collection strategies namely, how your concepts will be operationalized and the validity and reliability of your strategy. These concepts will be explored in the following section in the context of qualitative data gathering, and then specific sources of qualitative data will be discussed.

KEY CONCEPTS TO CONSIDER WHEN GATHERING QUALITATIVE DATA

Defining key concepts

Defining your key concepts or variables is a crucial step in the data-gathering process. First, nominal or dictionary type definitions are established, whereby you assert your theoretical understanding of the key concepts in your study. For example, if you are studying child–caregiver attachment you would assert not only what you mean by attachment (what theoretical understanding of attachment do you hold and what its key dimensions are), but also what you mean by "child" (are you looking at specific ages, biological children, foster-children, etc.?) and caregiver (how do you establish criteria that determines caregiver, is it hours per week spent with the child, is it a biological parent, an adoptive parent, a kin-foster-parent, etc., or other criteria?) In this way you are setting clear parameters for your qualitative study and ensuring that someone else could apply the same criteria to replicate your study if they wished. Or, they might replicate it with a different population, for example from a different cultural group, for comparative purposes.

Once you have established your nominal definitions then you must operationalize your key concepts. The operational definition of a concept refers to the exact way in which the concept will be measured. This process of "operationalization", while more commonly associated with quantitative data, is equally crucial for qualitative studies. It is imperative that you know how you will ask your questions or frame your observations, what criteria you will use to identify key concepts within the study, and how you will code or classify specific qualitative responses or observed behaviors. What differs, is that in quantitative data gathering both the questions and the potential response categories are constructed before data are collected. In qualitative data gathering, the questions are pre-set but the answer categories are derived from the responses themselves.

So, for example, in our quantitative study of depression in the previous chapter (using Box 6.1 on page 80), we operationalized depression using one of the existing standardized scales in which both questions and response categories were already established. Then we collected data and scored it based on the data we collected and norms that had been established with other populations with which the instrument had been used in prior studies.

As a practitioner-researcher conducting a qualitative study of depression, however, you may operationalize depression by using a clinical assessment of symptoms you observed in a client's behavior or responses that a client gave you to open-ended questions that you routinely ask in an intake interview. Then you might interpret behaviors observed, and/or interview responses to patterns that you already recognize as indicative of depression, or you might use the DSM-IV-TR criteria for major depressive disorder or some other symptom criteria to determine level of depression manifested by your client (APA, 2000). You might also want to decide what criteria you would use to designate mild, moderate, or severe depression. Working together, for example, in a school-based program for adolescents with other social workers, you might want to develop a protocol for conducting the assessments so that you can all agree on qualitative indicators and clusters of indicators of different degrees of depression in the young people with whom you are all working. Once done, ideally, you would double check to see that you and each of your social work team members who are conducting assessments are using similar criteria in their subsequent assessments. Likewise, if you were doing a retrospective, qualitative data-mining study using available data from case records, you would want to be sure that the same criteria for recognizing and rating depression had been used by all parties involved in data collection.

This concept of checking that there is a high level of agreement (80 percent or better) and application of criteria among all clinicians is referred to as inter-rater reliability. Similarly, if one were conducting the PBR study solo, the same principles would be used to monitor intra-rater reliability to ensure that the PBR researcher was applying assessment criteria consistently across cases.

In qualitative data gathering, reliability refers to the extent to which your coding procedure yields consistent results. So, it is important to establish that the criteria used to classify or score the data are employed consistently. If you are gathering qualitative data by data mining client records, and you are doing the data extraction it is essential that you are consistent in your coding over time. Thus, if based on the record you code a client at intake as being "moderately depressed", it would be important that the coding instructions you are following are precise enough for you to code that person as "moderately depressed" if you reviewed the same case on a different day. This is an even more refined application of the concept of intra-rater reliability than if you were simply determining whether a client is depressed or not.

Similarly, if you are working with others in a data-mining study, instructions for coding must be clear enough for all of the other data-extractors to be consistent in their coding of the same sets of symptoms for all client records. Concern about this form of consistency refers to the concept of inter-rater reliability mentioned above. In other words, if presented with the same case record, every data-extractor should code that client "moderately depressed" at intake. And, while it is unlikely that any individual will be totally consistent or any set of coders will have perfect agreement, there should be a very high degree of agreement for us to consider our coding "reliable". In quantitative data mining, statistical measures of reliability are employed. In qualitative data mining, while "reliability coefficients" aren't calculated, the same general principles apply.

If the validity of a measure in quantitative data gathering is the extent to which it measures what it is intended to measure, then in qualitative data gathering it is the extent to which your questions and the categories used to capture responses are directly relevant to the key concepts or dimensions about which your study is intended. So, the categories that you create as a means to understanding your data should be accurate and meaningful indicators of the concept that you are studying. While there are not specific validity tests for qualitative data as there are in quantitative data (see Chapter 8), you can apply the logic of face/content validity to judge whether "on the face of it" your questions, observations and the way you code responses are pertinent to the concepts you are studying.

So, for example, if you are doing family therapy and you employ the concept of "enmeshment", it will be extremely important to say what you mean by it when you observe it in family interviews. Equally, important is the ability to say when enmeshment is not present. Questions intended to reveal the presence or absence of enmeshment and responses to these questions need to be carefully considered for both clinical and research purposes.

Another key concept that is important in qualitative data gathering is triangulation, a technique that is frequently used in qualitative research to verify and validate inferences made from qualitative data. Triangulation involves gathering data about the same thing from different types of data sources to test the extent that the data gathered are or are not consistent. Very consistent data received from several different types of sources lend much stronger support to your findings than when inconsistent data patterns emerge from the different sources. Whether qualitative or quantitative data gathering, it is always preferable to gather data about key variables from multiple sources.

This is true in practice as well. For example, a social worker working with a depressed adolescent would ideally want to meet with parents/guardians and teachers as well as the young person to validly and reliably assess the problem. Perhaps the young person is witnessing violence in the home? Perhaps she or he has a learning disorder, or is being bullied in school on account of sexual orientation or ethnic background? Gathering information from multiple sources is obviously better than relying on one source alone.

Finally, data checking is another tool in qualitative research that is closely related to triangulation. It involves returning to the source of original data collection to see to it that you "got it right", that is that the interpretations and inferences that you made based on your original data collection and analysis were consistent with the intended meanings of the study participants. This concept resembles in some ways what clinicians do in exit interviews or perhaps during individual treatment sessions to validate their interpretations and to see whether they "square" with the client's perception and intended meaning. Often, from a psychological point of view, such efforts both "validate" clients' rights to their feelings as well as the expertise of the worker.

In an entirely different practice arena, nothing is as much a non-starter as a community organizer who does not correctly listen to and interpret back how the community initially defines its problem but then goes on to impose her or his own interpretation of what is "correct". In clinical, program and community organization efforts these things can change, but "starting where the client is" has always been a fundamental principle of social work practice. Data checking involves determining where they were when the data were collected.

All of the research concepts discussed above are as useful in practice as in research. The degree to which they are applied and quantified is a matter of style and convenience. In PBR, they are employed in ways that inform but are not imposed on practice.

PRACTICE PARALLELS IN QUALITATIVE DATA GATHERING

The NASW code of ethics highlights the value of human relationships, and almost all social work relies on interpersonal relationships as the mechanism for intervention (NASW, 2008). We engage with clients, groups, communities and agencies in order to establish relationships and develop trust in our efforts to create positive change. Similar characteristics are an essential feature as you begin to consider generating original qualitative data. The interaction between you the practitioner-researcher and the client-participant involves an interpersonal relationship, sometimes brief and sometimes longstanding. Rapport must be established in order to provide a safe and open context within which meaningful information can be shared. Through this rapport comes the development of trust, which stands at the cornerstone of observations and interviews (and, of course, good social work practice). The development of trust and rapport is also a key aspect in the retention versus attrition of your study participants. At the back of a participant's mind (or perhaps at the front) as they respond to interview questions or allow themselves to be videotaped is the question "what will you do with what I say?" (Matthews and Cramer, 2008). Therefore, as a practitioner-researcher you must be careful to clearly specify the purposes of your data gathering and work hard to avoid coercing your clients into participation. We explore the concept of research ethics more generally, and coercion in particular, as they apply to PBR in Chapter 10.

Power dynamics are central to all practice and to all research relationships. In RBP they are more straightforward though arguably potentially more coercive than in PBR. In PBR, however, power dynamics are subtler since PBR occurs most commonly in a practice setting where you the practitioner are in a professional relationship with clients and the client community. Hence, there is an added power dynamic inherent in attempting to combine practice and research. These power dynamics can influence not only the extent to which people choose whether or not to participate in a study (the coercion we referred to above), but also the type, quantity and quality of information that they share about themselves during the research. This can be especially true when gathering qualitative data where people are not following prescribed answer options, but rather are responding spontaneously to questions as they arise. As you would when following sound practice principles, you should make every effort to both acknowledge the power that you hold, and minimize the interference of that power by allowing the voice of the participant to come through loudly as a co-creator of the information (Loutzenheiser, 2007).

The seductive and vulnerable dynamic situation created by "being paid attention to" during the research process, has led to some participants acknowledging that they revealed "more than they wanted to" in interviews in an effort to act appropriately and provide the "right" answer (Beckett and Clegg, 2007, p.310). In that particular case, a study of sexual minority individuals, the authors decided that it was more ethical to interview oppressed groups asynchronously, that is not face-to-face, but rather using a written interview that allowed participants to reflect on their responses and choose the degree of disclosure that they are comfortable with before submitting their responses (Beckett and Clegg, 2007). So, bearing in mind the vulnerabilities of the population that you are studying, the potential for coercion, your explicit and implicit contract with them and the presence of varying power dynamics, the following data sources are available for you to select from when conducting a qualitative PBR study. Perhaps the most useful PBR principle to keep in mind, however, is don't do anything for research purposes that you wouldn't ordinarily do in practice. If you are in doubt, you can always consult with an agency or university-based human subjects or ethics committee. There is more about research ethics and practice in Chapter 10.

QUALITATIVE DATA SOURCES

There are different ways to generate original data or access available qualitative data (the same is true for quantitative data as you will see in the next chapter). Original or primary qualitative data sources may be generated by interviewing your client in person, on the telephone, via Skype (or other video-conferencing technology), or in written form; or by observing your client or specific events in person or via videotape.

Secondary data sources of qualitative data include existing documentation or videotapes that were generated for practice, research or for other purposes, but that are available for you to study. Examples of qualitative documents that may be available for you to study via secondary analysis include client case records, worker process recordings, minutes of meetings or agency policies. "Secondary analyses" are usually conducted with available databases intended for research, but not with your specific question in mind. Qualitative clinical data mining is a newly developing form of PBR that involves qualitative analysis of clinical data not originally intended for research purposes.

Interviews

There are a number of different ways to generate original qualitative data by interviewing participants about the topic that you are studying. Interviews can vary considerably in format, structure, and length. As you plan your PBR study you will have to make choices about the format that is most suitable for your study purpose based on the strengths and weaknesses of each option, your particular practice setting, and the people that you are studying. Should the interview be in person or use information technology? Will it involve an individual, family or group? Will it involve present clients, prospective clients or "key informants" who are especially knowledgeable about clients and/or the client community?

You also have to plan whether your interview will be highly structured following closely to a script or will it be guided by just a few open-ended questions that you follow wherever the respondent takes you? Finally, you will have to decide the appropriate length of the interview, balancing your need for information with your respondent's interest, intellectual capacity and health. The following sections explore some of the different options of format, structure, and length available to you.

In-person interviews are conducted in person, and so can offer the practitioner-researcher the advantage of observing non-verbal cues and body language as part of the interview process. Also, given the importance of establishing relationship, rapport, and trust, in-person interviews provide the advantage of allowing the practitioner-researcher and the participant(s) to "see" each other as a way of connecting. In-person interviews are more difficult to organize logistically because they are limited by geography, requiring the interviewer and interviewee to be in the same geographic location (as travel is both expensive and time-consuming). Technological advances have helped to erase some of these drawbacks.

Web camera interviews can provide the advantages of in-person, synchronous interviews without the drawbacks of limited geographic sample range, and the added cost of travel expenses and time. Of course, one inherent drawback of these is that both the interviewer and the interviewee must have access to and the capacity to successfully interact with a computer and webcam technology. Certainly technology is increasingly available but specific demographics of client populations (the elderly, those from lower socio-economic and educational backgrounds, and those disinclined to employ technology) may be excluded if webcam is the only method of interviewing used in the study. Such exclusion may limit the availability of study participants, and therefore your findings. Worse still, if availability is associated with the issue you are studying, your findings will be biased in one direction or another. So, for example, limiting interviews about future community center services to those who have access to Skype will very likely introduce both a social class and an age bias into your findings.

Since building trust and rapport are key factors in the success of interviews, and may also impact future program participation rates, it is very important to consider how you are presenting yourself for in-person interviews. Just as you would when following good practice principles, you should pay attention to the way in which you present yourself in the interview in a way that facilitates comfort on the part of the participant. You do not want to create distance by dressing in a way that will make participants uncomfortable by dressing too formally in a way that emphasizes a power differential. On the other hand, you do not want to dress so informally that you dilute your credibility and suggest a lack of respect for respondents.

Telephone interviews are a very popular way of reaching a diverse geographic set of respondents without adding travel expenses, the need for computers on the respondent's end or your need to find a private, neutral space for the interview. Though not as good as seeing the respondent, during telephone interviews you can still detect audible non-verbal cues, such as hesitations, pauses, coughs or laughs, but you obviously cannot detect any visual cues. While many more people have access to a telephone than to a webcam, some people will still be excluded from your study because they do not have access to a telephone or because they are unavailable when you call. Providing phone cards for payphones or "minutes" for cell phone plans can increase the potential participant pool.

Focus groups

Focus groups are a special kind of in-person interview that gather qualitative data from small groups rather than individuals. The selection of participants for focus group interviews usually involves people who share similar social characteristics or common experiences about which they are treated as "experts". Focus group participants can come together around any unifying topic, for example they may all be GLBT parents of young children, caregivers of parents with Alzheimer's in the "sandwich" generation, previously unemployed people who have received employment counseling services from a particular service provider, or teens attending an after-school program whose parents have divorced.

As indicated above, the major attraction of using a focus group to collect qualitative data is that you can get feedback from a number of people at the same time and you can quickly get a sense of the extent to which a range of people agree or disagree about a point. The advantage of focus groups is not only economy (i.e. more respondents per interview) but the opportunity for respondents to interact and provoke richer and deeper responses from each other. On the other hand, depending on how sensitive the topic, some respondents will only reveal things about themselves in in-person, one-on-one interviews. Still, the efficiency and depth of data provided in skillfully-run focus groups is one of the reasons that politicians and the social workers who work for them use focus groups to gather feedback from different constituent groups, so that they can make legislative and policy decisions.

While focus groups have many advantages they also have some disadvantages. For example, a drawback of focus groups is that participants may be influenced by the sentiment of the group. Participants may provide socially acceptable responses or answers consistent with those that they think are expected by the group. Often in groups there can be a dominant personality, who may influence the direction of the conversation, with quieter or less forceful personalities being pulled along by the crowd or limiting their participation in the dialogue. Skillful focus group facilitation involves allowing the conversation to flow while trying to pull in the different voices that may be present in the room and testing the group's consensus around the validity of the statements being made from their experience. Like a skillful group worker, a skillful focus group facilitator is sufficiently mindful and in control of her or his own verbal interventions and body language so as not to unduly influence the direction of the dialogue or imply that some responses are more acceptable than others.

Interview structure

Interviews and interview guides have varying degrees of structure depending on the state of the knowledge about the subject of the interview and sometimes the interviewer's "style". Here again, as in social work practice, the style of the interview should match the study purpose and the respondent's needs rather than the interviewer's preferences.

Structured interviews have a clear and concise "guide" or "script" with specific questions and a logical order that is followed faithfully by the interviewer with pre-designated "probes" (e.g. "can you say more about that?") to use when the respondent draws a blank or gives shallow, automatic or even seemingly inauthentic responses. Because the questions are constructed beforehand, any data gathered are inevitably shaped by the practitioner-researcher's notions about the topic being studied (Goodman, 2001). At the other end of the interview spectrum are unstructured interviews whereby the interviewer has few preconceived questions and no particular order to follow. Probes are employed but not pre-selected. Leaving the interview unstructured or open-ended allows the practitioner-researcher to keep their notions about a topic out of the way. However, open-ended interviews rely heavily on the capacity of the interviewer to be fully present and to operate reflectively throughout the interview, creating questions that can help to support or dispute what may already be known about a topic (Goodman, 2001). Clearly, such an interview resembles clinical practice in many ways. The differences are that an RBP interview is primarily intended to gather research-relevant information, a PBR interview is intended to gather practice-relevant research information and a clinical interview is intended to gather practice-relevant information with research absent from the agenda.

In-depth or semi-structured interviews fall somewhere between these two extremes. The interviewer starts with some broad topical questions that they intend to ask, and they have systematic probes outlined to ensure that key areas get covered. But the interview is structured more like a conversation so that the interviewer may switch the order in which topics are pursued in order to maintain the ease and flow of the interaction. In many ways the semi-structured interview mirrors the process used by social workers during an intake assessment, where key content areas need to be covered but not necessarily in a specific order. Skilled social workers will follow up on content that they think important and possibly relevant to the case, before moving on to a new topic. Focus groups most often follow the semi-structured format since it allows for dialogue to occur between group members and can use the energy of the group and group discussion to dictate the order of the topics being covered.

Synchronous interviews are those that occur in real time either in-person, by phone, via a web-based instant messaging system or via a webcam such as Skype or iChat. A key advantage to synchronous interviews is that the interviewer can ask for clarification of a particular point or restate information to check that it was properly understood. By contrast, asynchronous interviews are those that do not happen in "real time". The interview may be mailed or emailed with respondents answering in their own time. Most often the interaction involves a one-time response, but in other formats the questions and responses go back and forth as in a chat-room. When responses are single shot only, then the interviewer loses the opportunity to probe deeper into a particular answer or to ask for clarification concerning a particular response though these are more efficient for the researcher and less burdensome to the respondent – unless of course the respondent is thoroughly engaged in the topic and looks forward to an in-depth exchange.

For a long time it was thought that synchronous interviews were most effective since they allowed the interviewer to attend to the reactions and responses of the interviewee and to allow the interview to unfold through shared interaction. The interview setting was thought to create a climate of "intimacy and authenticity" (Beckett and Clegg, 2007, p.308). However, as we mentioned earlier, it has been suggested that at least for some oppressed groups asynchronous non-present interviews allow participants the time and opportunity to reflect on their degree of disclosure, and presents a climate of "safety", which produces more authentic "data" (Beckett and Clegg, 2007).

Interview length

Interviews range from very brief to very long. The purpose of the interview should be central to determining the length, as should the functioning level of the participant. A two-question poll may take just a few minutes whereas a detailed clinical interview may take a few hours. As with questionnaires, interviews should be as short as possible while asking all the questions needed to gather the relevant information. Whatever the purpose, structure or length of the interview however, attention should be paid to avoid extraneous questions that may be of tangential interest but are not central to the purpose of the particular practice-based research question.

Children, especially young children, have a lower capacity to sit still and concentrate for long periods of time than most adults, so interviews with children should be short or punctuated with active breaks. The same may be true for older adults or people with serious medical conditions; they may get tired if the interview continues for too long without a break. Focus groups tend to be a little longer than interviews, since you are trying to allow time for multiple people to express their opinions. So, it is not uncommon for a focus group to run for an hour and a half or even longer and to provide food and beverages as a reward beforehand. While some researchers provide food and drinks after as a thank you, providing food beforehand can serve the useful purpose of giving participants an opportunity to become familiar with each other before the interview takes place.

Observations

Qualitative data generated via observations can occur live, via videotape or both. When conducting live observations the role of the observer can vary from passive non-participant, through partial participation, to full participation (known as being a participant-observer). The observer's role may also be known or unknown to those being observed. Whether or not you are a participant-observer, when generating data via observation it is common to take field notes to describe what you are observing or to record your thoughts into a handheld tape recorder. Without some way to capture your observations as they occur, you are reliant on your memory to accurately recall what you witnessed. For an especially exciting and complex observation this can be a particular challenge (or for those of us of advanced age!) In ethnographic research conducted by anthropologists the intention generally is to faithfully describe and understand the dynamics of the group or culture being studied but to scrupulously avoid changing it. Sometimes the latter can't be helped such as when cultural groups under study are exposed for the first time to computers or cell phones or phones that take pictures. In PBR observation research, change is an acceptable option especially when those observed are requesting assistance.

While an important advantage of observations is that they allow the researcher to witness behavior and dynamics within their real-world natural setting, a disadvantage is that it is possible for the very act of observation to obscure the behavior being observed, by creating what is called reactivity. Reactivity refers to the extent that those being observed have a reaction to being observed which causes them to adjust their behavior in some way. Just as students in a classroom may suddenly become quiet and "well-behaved" when a principal walks in, so a family may adjust its dynamics to what it perceives is "appropriate behavior" when a family therapist or protective service worker begins his or her observation of their dinnertime ritual or merely conducts a home visit. Still, it is clear that home visits provide so much more understanding of family and parent–child dynamics than do office visits alone.

Structured observations are those where a particular type or pattern of behavior is observed and recorded. In qualitative observation research, data are collected in words and possibly pictures and moving images. In quantitative observation research, behaviors are counted and recorded. More structured observations can record the number of times a particular event occurs, e.g. the number of times a teacher calls on male students versus female students or attends to positive academic versus negative breaches of "comportment" (Epstein and Hench, 1979), or the number of times a parent uses positive reinforcement versus punitive responses while helping a child do homework. By contrast, unstructured observations tend to generate qualitative data that is focused more on patterns and themes of behaviors that emerge. Unstructured observations are more commonly used when very little is known about a topic and you are trying to gather preliminary data to begin to conceptualize the issue.

Whatever the form of observation, it is important to be thoughtful about the timing of observations, specifying exactly when they will occur. Will observations occur for one hour at the same time every morning for a week, or will observation times vary in an attempt to discern patterns that may differ at different times of the day. However, here again as with other PBR data-collection strategies, observations should be as unobtrusive as possible so as to not compromise practice and program purposes. This is about research in practice rather than research on practice.

CONTENT ANALYSIS, SECONDARY ANALYSIS AND QUALITATIVE CDM

Content analysis

Content analysis is the general term that researchers use to analyze data from existing documents, such as case records, agency policy documents, meeting minutes, or written narratives. Such studies often involve counting the number of key words or significant phrases used in existing qualitative data sources. The goal in content analysis is to identify themes and patterns that are present within a set of documents, electronic posts, pictures, or movies. The process of content analysis utilizes a coding scheme that establishes exhaustive and mutually exclusive categories just as you would when establishing nominal level quantitative data (see Chapter 11). The CIA for example uses computer programs that scan emails between suspected terrorists to identify key words or phrases that might indicate future national security threats. While we are all for national security, we anticipate that you will find a more pedestrian use of research and research ways of thinking to enhance your practice and service to clients and the community.

Secondary analysis and CDM

Secondary analysis is a term generally used to describe quantitative analysis or available quantitative data that was originally collected and intended for research purposes. By contrast, clinical data mining (CDM) is a term we use to describe the analysis of available clinical or program data that was not originally intended for research. At most the latter was intended for accountability purposes. But CDM involves collecting these data and using them for PBR purposes.

In the next chapter we will explore how CDM might involve collecting and quantitatively analyzing data that is already in quantitative form such as client intake data or numbers of treatment sessions or outcome data such as is available in client satisfaction survey data. Other CDM studies involve converting originally qualitative data (such as client process records) into quantitative data and analyzing it as such. Here in some respects, CDM parallels content analysis though its purposes are either clinical or programmatic.

While some CDM studies may leave the data in qualitative form, others may transform available qualitative data into quantitative form keeping tallies perhaps of the number of times a particular diagnosis appears in the client population, or the number of times a specific referral is made. The conversion of qualitative data into quantitative data is quite common in clinical data-mining studies. This process of data conversion involves the creation of a data-extraction instrument that looks very much like a quantitative questionnaire, which follows the same principles but is used to "interrogate" the case record. To conduct CDM ethically, data sets are easily "de-identified" so that the raw data and study findings cannot be linked to particular clients, patients or their families. However, no magic software has yet been devised, which can convert quantitative available data into qualitative data (perhaps by the 10th edition of this book this will be possible).

Qualitative CDM involves collecting available qualitative data and analyzing it qualitatively (Epstein, 2010). Qualitative CDM can be extremely informative depending on the richness and "thickness" of the available data source. So, for example, Jones, Statham and Solomou (2006) have conducted a psycho-dynamically insightful study of the clinical needs of women who are going through with pregnancies with a known fetal abnormality rather than seeking abortion. Based on a sample of only 7 women in this difficult and complex situation, the feasibility of their study was contingent on the richness of interview data available from the discovery of the abnormality through and after the birth of the child.

In the first qualitative CDM doctoral dissertation that we know of, Cordero conducted a study of social work practice that promoted successful foster-care reunification (Cordero, 2000). The study described in rich detail, problems and interventions with foster parents, biological parents and children at various stages in the casework process – from initial placement to return home. Though conducted with a relatively small sample of 19 successful cases, Cordero's qualitative CDM study was only possible because of the detailed process records available at the foster-care agency in which she conducted it.

SUMMARY OF KEY CONCEPTS

In this chapter we explored a range of concepts relevant to qualitative data gathering. First, we indicated the ways in which nominal and operational definitions, and reliability and validity applied within the context of qualitative data gathering. We then explored potential sources of qualitative data, including different interview formats, focus groups and observations noting the strengths and weaknesses of each source. We discussed the merits of synchronous versus asynchronous interviews and finally we reviewed content analysis of secondary data sources. The following chapter will explore many of these same concepts as they relate to quantitative data gathering.

Chapter 8

Quantitative data gathering

Purpose

Having introduced you to qualitative data-gathering strategies in the last chapter, this chapter focuses on quantitative data gathering, i.e. data collected numerically and analyzed statistically. Key concepts relevant to quantitative data collection and the way in which practice-relevant concepts are "measured" will be explored, as will sources of quantitative data. Combining qualitative and quantitative approaches into a mixed-methods approach will also be discussed.

INTRODUCTION

Despite the advent of user-friendly statistical software programs, many social work students and practitioners shy away from quantitative studies because of their fear of statistics (Harder, 2010). This is unfortunate since quantitative studies can tell us a great deal and, for better or for worse, they represent the dominant form of published academic research in social work. Consequently, any meaningful review of the research literature for RBP or for PBR purposes requires a basic understanding of quantitative methods of data collection, analysis and interpretation.

CONCEPTS TO CONSIDER WHEN GATHERING QUANTITATIVE DATA

In this section we revisit many of the concepts we explored relative to qualitative data gathering, only now as they apply to quantitative data. When engaging in PBR and selecting your data sources there are some central research questions that need to be considered. The first, is exactly what are you going to study and how do you define key concepts that are central to your study question? The second is how do you know whether the measure you use accurately reflects the concepts that you are intending to study? The third is are you consistent in your measurement of these concepts? And the fourth is how refined will be the data that you are gathering and the analysis you are employing?

The specific research concepts and techniques used to help us answer these questions are operationalization, validity, reliability, and level of measurement respectively. The following section considers (or reconsiders) each of these quantitative research questions and the tools researchers use to answer them.

DEFINING KEY CONCEPTS

As with qualitative data, in doing quantitative research on any particular dimension, you begin by precisely defining the key concepts in the study. As you will recall, nominal definitions of your concepts are established during the problem formulation phase. Nominal definitions describe what you mean by each concept using words in much the same way your dictionary does. However, as you move on to plan your data-collection strategy you also need to establish the exact way in which the concepts will be quantitatively measured. This is known as their operational definition. If you are constructing a self-administered questionnaire for example, it means what specific questions you will ask to measure each important concept, what the answers might be and how those responses will be numerically scored.

Revisiting our depression study as an example, as a practitioner-researcher utilizing quantitative methodology and employing a standardized instrument you would need to operationalize depression, that is you would need to specify exactly which of the available scales you are going to use or adapt to measure depression. Or, you might develop your own.

One advantage of using a pre-existing scale is that someone else has already operationalized the specific questions and scoring procedures and even established "norms" about how people respond so that they might be reliably labeled "extremely", "moderately" or "slightly" depressed or "not depressed" at all. Still, in studying dimensions like depression where many scales exist, you would still have to decide which one to use.

To do this, you would look at the attributes of the scales and the populations they are designed for, you would consider the number of questions and the way in which the scale is administered and then make your selection. You might choose the Hamilton Rating Scale for Depression (Hamilton, 1980), or the Beck Depression Inventory (Beck *et al.*, 1996), or if you are working with older adults, the Geriatric Depression scale

(Yesavage *et al.*, 1983) which does not include questions about physical symptoms of depression that are skewed negatively for older adults. Once you have decided on which depression scale you will use then you need to be clear about the scoring method and the score thresholds that you will use to classify participants as mildly, moderately, or severely depressed.

When deciding on the most appropriate scale to use it is also important to consider how faithfully and completely it measures the concept that you are interested in studying. We call this measurement validity. You also want to know the extent that the measure can consistently distinguish differences in the concept you are measuring, we call this its reliability. The next two sections will explore these two research concepts in greater detail.

Validity

Simply stated, the validity of a measure refers to the extent to which it measures what it is intended to measure. Accordingly, sometimes researchers talk about whether the concept (e.g. patient optimism) is directly reflected in the "indicators" used to measure it. Thus, if a patient is classified as optimistic about medical treatment because she or he says things that directly express optimism or chooses response options that indicate optimism, you are on safer ground than using indirect indicators such as patient affect (e.g. smiling) or adherence with physician recommendations about taking medications. Though the latter indicators might be indirectly associated with optimism, they are not the same thing. Smiling might indicate stoic denial and total compliance might indicate intense fear of a negative outcome.

There are different types of validity that can be established. Perhaps the easiest is face validity, which simply asserts that on the face of it the items on a scale or the criteria that you are using for coding are logically and directly related to the concept being measured. Thus, if asking a patient whether s/he was optimistic about the outcome of a medical procedure, an affirmative response would certainly satisfy our simplest criterion. An extension of face validity is content validity, which is established by asking "experts" whether they think the scale items or coding criteria capture the concept being measured. These experts might recommend changes, omissions and deletions in questions asked and in the numerical coding of different responses. Thus, response categories could range from "very optimistic" to "very pessimistic".

Another type of validity, criterion validity refers to the extent to which the results of your scale are consistent with criteria that distinguish your concept. There are two types of criterion validity – concurrent validity and predictive validity. In concurrent validity the scale is measured against an existing and established set of current criteria for the concept you are measuring. Thus, if you used the crudest, single question, "Yes"/"No" response measure, establishing concurrent validity would involve comparison of that simple question and response to a standardized measure of patient optimism to see the extent that the scores concur (agree). Thus, individual scores on that optimism question should predict scores on the existing criteria. Validity is established by showing a strong percentage agreement or correlation (80% or .80 or higher, respectively) between scores on the original scale and a scale that has already been developed by researchers to measure the same concept.

A drawback of this type of validity is that it is contingent on the validity of the comparison scale. This is why it is important to closely consider the content of the questions and response categories on standardized scales rather than to accept them at face-value, just because the scale is labeled what you are hoping to measure.

In predictive validity the scale score is measured against some criterion or criteria in the future. For example, the scholastic aptitude tests, the SAT, the LSAT and the GRE are supposed to determine scholastic aptitude for college, law school and graduate school respectively. Therefore, participant scores can be compared against their GPAs to see the extent to which their test scores predicted their future academic success. Sometimes a particular type of predictive validity called known-groups is used to validate a scale. An example of establishing known-groups validity would be if you have a group of participants that you know are accessing mental health services for trauma symptoms and a group that are not, then utilizing your trauma symptom scale you should be able to predict which participants belong to which group.

Construct validity is thought to be the highest and most conceptually "robust" form of validity and is tied to the theoretical framework of the concept being measured. Construct validity is related to the extent that you can determine whether all theoretical aspects of the concept are captured by the scale. Hence patient optimism might involve anticipation of future improved or restored functioning in multiple aspects of life as well as in a general way.

Convergent validity overlaps with concurrent validity and is specifically related to the extent to which scores between the scale being tested and an established scale measuring the same or similar concepts converge or overlap. By contrast, discriminant validity is established by comparing participant's scores on scales that look similar in terms of format, but that measure different concepts, i.e. the scales can discriminate between different concepts. For discriminant validity a low correlation score between two scales that measure different concepts supports validity. So scale scores should correlate or converge with related concepts and not correlate or diverge from unrelated concepts. While each of the foregoing involves a different approach to establishing validity, they all share the same general purpose, which is to assure that you are measuring what you intend to measure.

Reliability

Reliability as we indicated earlier, refers to the extent to which a measuring instrument, rating scale or coding procedure is applied consistently and yields consistent results. We introduced the concept in reference to inter- and intra-rater reliability in the previous chapter. When utilizing quantitative scales, there are two aspects of reliability to consider – stability and equivalence. If a measure is stable then it should not change from one application to the next, unless the variable being measured has actually changed. So, if your client is moderately depressed and hasn't changed from one assessment to another, it would be important that scoring procedures be such that the client would continue to be assessed as "moderately depressed".

In a very different but illustrative example, imagine if a client, Andy, were to step on a weighing scale and weighed 184 pounds, if he stepped off the scale and then immediately back on, one would assume that the subsequent reading would still be 184 pounds assuming he hadn't taken off his shoes. If he hadn't but the subsequent reading was 165 pounds, one would conclude that the weighing scale is "unstable", and therefore not reliable.

Equivalence, on the other hand, refers to the extent to which all items on a scale measure the same thing. So, for example, on a self-administered depression scale questions and responses about sleep patterns (when and how long?) might indicate depression for younger clients but something very different for older clients. Thus, a depression scale that relied heavily on questions about sleep would not have equivalence for adolescents or for retirees.

There are different statistical procedures for testing the reliability of quantitative measures including test–retest, multiple forms, and the split-half approach. In test–retest the instrument is administered to a particular group of clients and then re-administered to the same group of clients. However, the test and the retest have to be timed far enough apart so that people don't recall the answer they chose last time and repeat it, but not so far apart that the person has actually shifted on the dimension being measured. If the instrument is reliable and the respondents haven't changed then they should score similarly roughly 80 percent of the time. As we did for validity, in statistical terms we say that the two scores that are recorded should correlate to .80 or higher in order to establish reliability (stability) for the instrument. (Again, the statistical explanation behind correlations will be explored in Chapter 12.)

Multiple-forms reliability is established by creating two or more versions of the same scale. The logic behind multiple forms is that respondents' scores on two different versions of the same scale should be very similar if measured at the same point in time. Here again, reliability is established if the two forms correlate at a rate of .80 or higher. However, since generating one rating scale is already hard and generating more than one is twice as hard, then split-half reliability is a possible alternative. As its name implies, in split-half reliability, items on a scale are randomly divided in half to create two sub-scales out of the original one. As with multiple-forms reliability, participants are asked to complete both sub-scales and their scores on each are compared. Each individual's score on one sub-scale should correspond to their score on the other sub-scale. Again, a correlation of .80 is seen as the threshold of acceptable reliability for the total scale.

Another measure using the .80 criterion is the Cronbach Alpha score which measures the degree to which responses to single questions within the scale are internally consistent with all other items in every possible combination. But don't worry there are relatively simple computer programs to do all those calculations and to tell you which items don't work well when you are developing original scales. The importance of doing that is so that unreliable items can be dropped in order to increase the reliability of those remaining (see Weinbach and Grinnell, 2010; Craft, 1990 for further explanation).

Because most practitioners are neither inclined nor in a position to invest extensive time and resources into establishing the statistical reliability of the instruments they might use, practitioner-researchers are better off using pre-existing instruments in which reliability has already been established. However sometimes such instruments do not exist or the ones that do are too cumbersome and burdensome to administer with service recipients (Epstein, 2001). In such instances, the practitioner-researcher needs to develop her/his own measures, employing the underlying principle of reliability in instrument construction even though statistical testing is not feasible.

As with validity, academic researchers are content with reliability scores of .80 or better. However, it is important to be clear that validity and reliability are not the same thing. Thus, measures can be reliable (i.e. consistently applied) but not valid (i.e. unreflective of the concept they are intended to measure). So for example, if we were to "measure" social work student intelligence based on whether they wore glasses or not our measure would be fairly reliable but invalid. If we also knew which students wore contact lenses our measure would be even more reliable but still invalid.

Levels of measurement

A final important concept related to quantitative measurement is level of measurement. When collecting and analyzing quantitative data there are different ways to ask a question and to assign numbers to the answers. These differences importantly influence how you can statistically analyze the data and how you can present and interpret your findings (see the summary in Box 8.1).

So, for example, when asking about client age you may ask how old they are in years. This would give you a specific number representing each client's age. In analyzing the data for all clients you can, among other more refined statistical calculations, report the average age of your client population. If instead you ask clients to check boxes with 5-year age intervals, for example: 20–24, 25–29, 30–34, 35–39, etc., you may then report the percentage of all clients that fall into each age grouping but you can't report the average age. Should you decide to report the age distribution in 10-year intervals, as 20–29, 30–39, 40–49, you could still do this by recombining the data within the previous 5-year categories. However, if you began by collecting data in 10-year intervals you couldn't then report it in more specific 5-year categories.

Note, however, that if you ask the age question in an ungrouped way, you can do both. Should you make the mistake of designating groups as 20–25, 25–30, 30–35, etc. as a remarkable number of first-time questionnaire constructors have done, you can't say anything about client age because all the categories overlap. (Think about it but don't do it.)

Finally, how the response categories are organized will determine the kinds of statistical analysis you can employ in relating age to other variables such as presenting problem, services needed and received and treatment outcomes. Each of these considerations about how to collect and organize quantitative data refers to what we call level of measurement.

When developing a quantitative data-gathering strategy (either choosing an existing instrument or creating your own or some of both), it is important to consider the level of measurement of the data that you will be gathering. Since, the level of measurement determines the degree of sensitivity of statistical tests that can be employed, it is important to collect data at the highest level of measurement possible, unless it would be invasive or disruptive in practice to do so. Remember however, as in our age example, the level of measurement can always be collapsed down a level (i.e. fewer response categories) but never up a level (i.e. more response categories). So, you can move from a more precise measure to a less precise one for analysis purposes, but not vice versa.

There are four levels of measurement – nominal, ordinal, interval, and ratio (easy to remember if you speak French as the first letter for each level spells noir or black).

Still there is no magic (black or otherwise) in understanding this essential set of quantitative principles.

Nominal data reflect the lowest and "crudest" level of measurement, followed by ordinal, then interval, with ratio as the highest. Nominal data categorize facts in categories that are assigned arbitrary numbers, which do not indicate any rank order for that variable. So for example, we may categorize a client as male or female and for analytic purposes assign the number 1 to male and 2 to female, but not imply that women are more of anything than men in doing so. We might just as easily assign 1 to women and 2 to men without implying that women were less of anything than men. In other words, with nominal data, the numbers assigned have no intrinsic significance. Computer analysis of the data requires that numbers be assigned to response categories. (Patriarchal statistical convention usually attributes 0 to female and 1 to male for analysis purposes, but that discussion will be saved for a different book.)

Another simple key for constructing and understanding nominal data is that response categories must be both mutually exclusive and exhaustive. By the former is meant that they cannot overlap as in our 20–25, 25–30, 30–35 example. In well-designed nominal categories, respondents can be assigned or assign themselves to one and only one of the response categories offered. Additionally, the categories must exhaust the range of possibilities. With age for example, response categories must include every possible age which is why the highest age category might be "100 or above". With our example of gender, only providing the two options of male and female is very limiting for those who identify as transgender or gender queer, so it is important to try to fully exhaust possible responses in your list of answer options so as not to alienate a potential respondent. This is also why so many questionnaire items have an "other (write in) _____" category for responses that the researchers have not anticipated.

Ordinal data represent the next higher level of measurement wherein the numbers assigned to response categories reflect an intentional rank ordering from "lower" to "higher" on some specified dimension. Response categories must still be mutually exclusive and exhaustive but the numbers assigned for analytic purposes are no longer arbitrary. An example of an ordinal question might be "to what extent do you agree with the statement 'all social work practitioners should actively engage in PBR'" with " strongly agree", "agree", "neither agree nor disagree", "disagree", and "strongly disagree" as conventional "Likert scale" response options. These responses can be "rank ordered" in that we know where each one is in relation to each other one on a variable dimension we might label "favorability toward PBR". Recognizing that a "strongly agree" is most favorable and "strongly disagree" is least, we might assign categories from 5 to 1 to the respective categories reflecting their intended rank ordering. Or, we could assign them from 1 to 5, with a high score indicative of "opposition to PBR".

If you were asked to respond to this item before and after reading this book, our hope is that you would have scored a neutral "3" when you began and finished with a higher score on favorability or a lower score on opposition to PBR depending upon what rank ordering system we chose. But where you actually began and end remains an empirical question – the answer to which requires evidence.

Rank ordering allows you to do more sophisticated data analysis with ordinal data than with nominal data. However, ordinal data still have their limitations. Thus while you know where each response category ranks in "favorability" you can't say whether the intervals between each category are equivalent. Hence, you don't know whether the difference between a highly sophisticated student like yourself who strongly agrees with PBR favorability statements and someone who merely agrees (like your less sophisticated classmates) is as great as the difference between those "reluctants" who disagree and the "recalcitrants" who strongly disagree. Still, for computer analysis you could have just as easily assigned a number 4 to "strongly agree" and 0 to "strongly disagree". Thus the actual numbers assigned remain somewhat arbitrary and only have significance to the extent that they reflect a system of ranking.

Interval data differ from ordinal and nominal data because they have a numeric representation that carries a commonly shared meaning and cannot arbitrarily be changed. Response categories are still mutually exclusive and exhaustive and they are ranked, but now the numeric representation of the categories has intrinsic meaning and cannot be arbitrarily changed. In addition, for interval level data each category on the category continuum is presumed to be equidistant from the category preceding it or following it.

Take, for example, the frequently used Global Assessment of Functioning (GAF) scale used by mental health clinicians and physicians to rate the social, occupational, and psychological functioning of adults i.e. how well or adaptively one is meeting various problems-in-living (APA, 2000). GAF scores range from a possible 0 to 100 and the scale produces interval level data. Consequently, clients scoring 80 on a GAF score compared to clients scoring 70 are considered as different from each other as those scoring 42 and 32 respectively. And both clinicians and researchers who routinely employ the GAF have a general sense of what a score of 80 means as compared to a 70 or a 90. More generally, with interval level data we are able to do simple addition and subtraction between scores and the differences are treated as intrinsically meaningful with one exception. More specifically on the GAF scale, each point on the scale is considered as one unit of better or worse functioning. The only exception is the starting point, which remains arbitrary. Thus while, in principle, a client could receive a GAF score of 0, the original designers of the GAF could have started with 1: in interval data, there is no "true zero" and the 0 starting point for the scale is arbitrarily placed.

Another example frequently used to explain this concept is temperature scales – Fahrenheit and centigrade are both interval level variables that have 0 placed arbitrarily on their scale. Despite this limitation, you will see in later chapters that you can do many more statistical analyses with interval level data than with nominal or ordinal data. For example you can compute both the average GAF score and the average age of your client population but you cannot compute their average gender or race (nominal) or their average social class or level of education achievement (ordinal).

Ratio data have all the attributes of an interval scale (i.e. categories are mutually exclusive, exhaustive, rank ordered and equidistant from each other) but they also have a "true" or absolute zero. So if you asked clients how much sleep they had the night before seeing you, they could meaningfully respond that they had no sleep at all. Here, the zero is intrinsically meaningful. This allows us to perform mathematical procedures with the scores such as addition, subtraction, multiplication, and division. In other words, if homeless shelter clients reported on the average 3.5 hours sleep in the shelter and clients in their own apartments reported an average of 7 hours, you could meaningfully claim that those who had their own apartments slept twice as much as those living in shelters.

A key point here is to be mindful of the level of measurement of the questions that you ask and the response categories that you provide in collecting quantitative data. Always try to create questions and response categories at the highest level of measurement that "works" for your practice and that makes logical sense. Most importantly, use questions and response categories that clients can relate to. Some variables, such as gender, sexual orientation, religion, ethnicity can only be measured at the nominal level. And it is quite possible to study the relationships between lower level data and higher level, for example, between gender (nominal) and hours of sleep (ratio) in shelters. Though you can do the most statistically with scales that are at the highest level of measurement, your findings will have no meaning if client responses are neither valid nor reliable. That road leads to meaningless number-crunching.

QUANTITATIVE DATA-GATHERING STRATEGIES

Standardized instruments

Among RBP researchers, the most preferred data sources associated with quantitative methods of data collection are standardized instruments, sometimes called scales or indexes such as the GAF scale. These instruments are referred to as "standardized" because they bring with them very explicit instructions about how to administer,

---

BOX 8.1   LEVELS OF MEASUREMENT

Nominal   Classifies observations into different mutually exclusive and exhaustive categories. However, the numbers assigned are arbitrary and have no meaning. For example, Democrat could be assigned 1 and Republican assigned 2 or vice versa without any impact on the outcome.

Ordinal   The observations are mutually exclusive, exhaustive, and have some rank-order to them. Scales with anchors are ordinal. For example, a question using strongly agree, agree, neither agree nor disagree, disagree or strongly disagree. Notice, however, that the anchors could be assigned 1 through 5 or 5 through 1 and the meaning would not change. This is because the order is relevant but the actual number is not.

Interval   The numbers on an interval scale represent their meaning. There is an equal distance between each notch on the scale. Temperature, where 10 degrees is the same distance from 5 degrees and 15 degrees, is interval level. (It does not have a true zero because both Fahrenheit and centigrade have different zeros.)

Ratio   Ratio is considered the highest level of measurement. Ratio is the same as interval level but with an absolute zero. Distance, age, hours traveled all have an absolute zero. Scores can be multiplied and divided.

---

score, and classify the quantitative data they generate. Consequently, wherever they are used their scores are viewed as comparable, without extraneous factors affecting their results. Eighth-grade IQ scores in one school are treated as comparable to eighth-grade I.Q. scores in another school even if average IQ scores differ in the two schools.

Developing standardized scales requires rigorous testing on multiple populations to see if different groups have different response patterns. For example, an anxiety scale may be tested on adolescents, college-age students, adults and the elderly to see whether the questions response patterns and scores differ. Similarly, a scale may be tested to see whether the questions' "make sense", are applicable and can be interpreted similarly across different racial, ethnic, and cultural groups. By administering the scale to different groups and analyzing the results, the authors of the scale can establish group norms against which the scores of study participants can be compared.

You can't take claims to standardization on face value however. One of us (Epstein) had the experience of attempting to apply a "standardized" family coping scale in a juvenile correctional setting. Upon closer examination many of the items assumed more family resources (e.g. ownership of a car) and different family composition (e.g. dual parent families) than was reflected in the client population. As a result, to be meaningfully interpreted scores had to be "re-normed" based on the scores within the largely African-American, low-income client population of the setting and could not be compared with scores on the 2,000 white, middle-class, Christian, dual-parent families on which he later learned that the instrument had been tested and normed.

Standardized instruments are often used to measure abstract concepts, by including multiple indicators of that concept. So, for example, in your very first research class as a social work student you may be nervous or anxious so you may have an increased heart rate, sweaty palms, or feel agitated. If this bundle of physical and emotional indicators was used to create an anxiety scale then someone who had a slow heart rate, non-sweaty palms, and felt calm would score low for anxiety whereas someone with a rapid heart rate, very sweaty palms, and a powerful feeling of agitation would score high for anxiety. In this way we create a scale that uses multiple indicators to serve as proxy measures of the concept that they are measuring.

When a series of indicators are combined together to generate a composite score then it creates a scale or an index. For example, the Beck Depression Inventory (Beck *et al.*, 1996) is a very well-known frequently-used, self-report scale comprised of 21 questions reflecting multiple, agreed-upon clinical indicators associated with depression, such as feeling sad, crying, feeling irritable, loss of appetite, loss of interest in sexual activity, and inability to sleep. The 21 questions each have four potential responses ranging from 0–3, thus creating a 63-point scale. Each of the 21 questions is related to a symptom that Beck felt to be an important indicator of depression.

If you are interested in locating a standardized scale either to use in a PBR study or to use as a foundation for creating your own instrument they can be easily located. First, there are collections of measuring instruments available that index the scales both by subject e.g. trauma, youth development, marital satisfaction, etc. and by author. These collections include information about test administration, scoring, reliability, validity, the groups that it has been tested on and any norms that have been established. See for example Fischer and Corcoran (2007) *Measures for Clinical Practice: A sourcebook*, currently in its 4th edition, or, Keyser and Sweetland (2004) *Test Critiques*. Many of the instruments found in these collections of instruments are also now available online, although some require a fee for use. A simple Google search for anxiety measures reveals a list of several possible scales, including those that distinguish between "state" (fleeting) and "trait" (chronic) anxiety, and a review of scales to measure each. Many online links to scales also contain information regarding their reliability and validity.

Another good way of identifying instruments is to look at instruments used by existing studies. When you conduct a review of the literature (see Chapter 5), you can identify instruments used by others to measure the concepts or variables that you are interested in measuring, ideally with client populations and in programs similar to yours. As you gather literature, you can see what populations the scale was used on and what the article's author had to say about the appropriateness, practicality, reliability, and validity of the scale. Keep in mind that for PBR studies the extent to which the scale seems to be compatible with practice is an especially crucial point to evaluate.

Survey instruments

Standardized instruments may or may not be congenial to your client population or the protocols practiced in your program. Therefore, modifying existing agency intake or evaluation forms to include the data you seek may be a strategic option you want to consider for PBR purposes. Alternatively, you may have to create an original survey instrument to collect original quantitative data at a single point in time. For this you may employ items and response categories used in available instruments even though they are not standardized scales. Why take the time to invent items and response categories about variables studied in other research efforts when you can make use of the work of others? The adaptation of existing instruments appropriately reduces the additive burden of research for practitioners. Just be sure to cite them in your future publications – borrowing isn't plagiarism as long as it's acknowledged. One thing to think about here however is that by keeping the questions and response categories the same as in other studies, you can compare your findings with theirs. Once you change wording, response categories and scoring procedures, you can no longer make meaningful comparisons with the findings of these previous studies.

If you choose to create a survey instrument for PBR purposes or are looking to adapt your intake or other existing form then here are some things to consider. Who is your intended respondent population? Are they clients? Parents of clients? Community residents? Practitioners serving your clients? Practitioners serving clients like your own? And so on. It is important to understand who you are going to be gathering data from so that you can develop questions appropriate to their reading level, and in language that is consistent for their age and culture. For example, one of the authors (Dodd) was conducting a program evaluation about the effectiveness of an after-school program and chose to use pictures of faces expressing a range of emotions that ranged from smiley to sad so as to guide the students as to the meaning of the answers on the question scale (see Figure 8.1 overleaf).

When generating questionnaire items for a survey you should also consider closely what the purpose of your questions is and what it is that you are hoping to do with the results. It's never enough to say "wouldn't it be interesting to know?" You need to be able to say "why" you want to know otherwise your instrument will quickly grow unmanageably long and unnecessarily complicated.

Where possible, generate the forms with other social work colleagues or those responsible for implementing them, or even a small group of the intended respondent

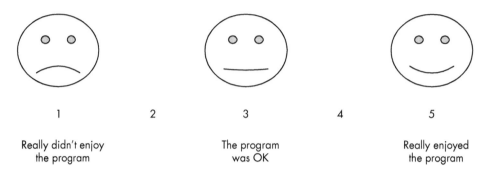

1   2   3   4   5

Really didn't enjoy   The program   Really enjoyed
the program   was OK   the program

FIGURE 8.1   Faces scale

population. At the very least, pre-test it with a few to get their feedback. You stand to gain a great deal from their expertise and familiarity with the issues in which you are interested while simultaneously generating feelings of ownership and their "buy-in" to the process on their part.

In one instance, a group of practitioners working in school-based mental health clinics across New York City worked together in collaboration with one of us to develop a survey to measure students' mental health, behavior, and academic status that could be used across all 5 clinics. The process facilitated both organizational learning and served as a learning tool for the practitioners (Dodd and Meezan, 2009; Cherin and Meezan, 1998). The dialogue that resulted created a supportive environ-ment for them to discuss similarities and differences across school environments and programs. The practitioners also successfully developed a PBR tool to track student progress as a means of evaluating their practice.

Boxes 8.2, 8.3 and 8.4 offer some general principles and specific suggestions about survey design and implementation that can help with survey development in terms of content, the construction of the actual questions, the response format of the questions and formatting in relation to how it appears to the respondent. These things signifi-cantly influence the rate at which people are likely to respond.

BOX 8.2   GENERAL PRINCIPLES FOR FORMATTING SURVEYS

1   Always give your survey a title – it orients the respondent.
2   Ensure that the language used matches your participants' level of compre-hension (or is translated into the appropriate language as needed).
3   Start with informed consent and a few clear instructions. Ensure that indi-viduals are informed fully of the uses of the information.
4   Keep questions as short as possible to keep the meaning clear.

Box 8.2 continued

5 Ask as few questions as possible to get the information you need (avoid asking unnecessary questions just out of interest). You should have a clinical or program-based reason to ask each question. "Wouldn't it be interesting to know?" Make sure that each question asks about only one issue and that response categories are mutually exclusive and exhaustive. If you can't anticipate all possible responses, include an "other (write in) _____" category.

6 Keep questions well spread – leave plenty of white space on a page

7 Use boxes, circles or numbers to allow for clear selection of choices.

8 Mix the slant of the questions to avoid response set; e.g. make some statements positive and some negative.

9 Always say "thank you" at the end.

BOX 8.3   SPECIFIC SUGGESTIONS FOR DEVELOPING SURVEYS

1 Start with interesting questions to grab the respondents' attention (put demographics at the end as they can put people off responding).

2 Put sensitive questions in the middle. Use clinical skills to develop forms that follow an arc from less intrusive questions to more intrusive/difficult questions then back to less intrusive.

3 Always capture the variable at the highest level of measurement unless it will have a very negative impact on the response rate (e.g. people are reluctant to report exact income but may be willing to check a box representing income range).

4 Never have a double-barrel question – it is not possible to answer honestly if the two choices conflict, e.g. if you ask "are you experienced and confident with SPSS?" Your respondent may be experienced but not confident.

5 For important variables have multiple items.

6 When possible use a mix of closed-ended and open-ended questions.

7 When selecting "anchors", i.e. numbers to which categories are assigned, try to make the anchors the same so that it is easy for the respondent to follow what they are answering, e.g. strongly disagree, disagree, etc.

8 Don't use a single format for questions and response categories throughout the survey (boring), but don't vary it so much that respondents spend more time reading instructions than answering questions (maddening).

9 Put very clear instructions, especially with contingency questions, e.g. "If you answer no, please go to Question 3. If yes, please go to Question 5".

BOX 8.4   ADDITIONAL SUGGESTIONS ABOUT SURVEY
IMPLEMENTATION

1 Always pilot test the questions to make sure that the questions are interpreted in the way that you would expect, to check that it was possible to
   follow your instructions, and to check that the answers you get allow you
   to answer your intended research question.
2 If you are using a web-based survey provider such as Survey Monkey,
   always take the test yourself before it goes live to check for any errors or
   missed questions. It is usually also good to take the test again as soon as it
   is live to check that there are no changes from the non-live practice run.

USING AVAILABLE QUANTITATIVE DATA

Some researchers and non-researchers alike think that the only way to conduct research is to collect original data via questionnaires, interviews, focus groups, direct observation, etc. While original data collection has real advantages because it can be targeted precisely to answer the research question that is driving the study, it has real disadvantages as well – particularly in PBR. The disadvantages of original data collection principally concern practice intrusiveness and time taken away from practice.

In other words, conducting a study based on original data often means disrupting routine practice protocols. For this reason, a guiding principle for the PBR-researcher should be that any data-collection strategy that involves original data collection should have a clinical or programmatic value as well as a research purpose. Thus, a questionnaire should do double duty as an intake or client satisfaction instrument as well as to generate research data. An interview at the end of treatment should help clients with the termination process as well as providing worker feedback. Focus groups should be used to reinforce resiliency and provide networking possibilities as well as offer new programmatic ideas.

So, it should be clear that to us, research and practice are compatible but not automatically. You've got to work at it. Like any partnership or marriage, compatibility requires intention and strategizing to make it happen. In RBP, clearly the preference is original data collection. In PBR, however, the starting point in thinking about data collection is available data. The obvious reason for this is that using data that is already there means no intrusion in or interruption of practice.

There are two kinds of research strategies employing available data – secondary analysis and clinical data mining. Secondary analysis involves analysis of data that has already been collected for research purposes (Sales, Lichtenwalter and Fevola, 2006). The data may have been collected already by a researcher who was studying a problem related to your practice interest and is willing to let you use the pre-existing data to explore your own interests. Harder (2010) describes how she makes agency-based data sets available to her MSW research students to neutralize their "reluctance" to studying research and to demonstrate how useful it can be for practice.

Alternatively, some RBP researchers purchase access to large, public-health oriented national databases which are specifically designed to promote research by multiple researchers in different locations. Examples might be the Centers for Disease Control (CDC) or the Substance Abuse and Mental Health Services Administration (SAMHSA). These databases are generally quantitative and often involve the use of standardized instruments of various kinds. Some of them are periodically replicated to allow for studying longitudinal trends in phenomena such as HIV-AIDS infections, suicide, mental hospitalization, etc. Although research with these large databases precludes the need for original data collection and has broad societal implications, most PBR researchers have neither access to them nor the kinds of skills required to statistically manipulate large data sets. However, some policy-oriented PhD programs in social welfare, public health and policy routinely teach doctoral students how to do so. Moreover, with some ingenuity, they can be used quite creatively to study highly relevant practice issues.

For his doctoral dissertation, Schmidt (2010), for example recently conducted a secondary analysis on the National Epidemiologic Survey on Alcohol and Related Conditions (NESARC), which involved a national sample of 34,653 men and women looking at discordant sexual identity (i.e. incongruence between one's self-definition of sexual attraction, sexual behavior, and sexual identity) and their HIV-related risk-taking. Not only was the conceptualization of this study ground-breaking, but the findings were quite surprising. Hence secondary analyses of existing databases can turn up highly relevant and unanticipated findings.

More suitable to practitioner-researchers at the MSW level as well as offering possibilities for doctoral dissertation research is clinical data mining (CDM). CDM involves the conceptualization, extraction, analysis and interpretation of routinely available data for practice knowledge-building, clinical decision-making and practitioner reflection (Epstein, 2010). Since social work, allied health and other human service professionals routinely generate and record enormous quantities of information concerning their clients, their interventions and the outcomes they either produce or do not produce, "mining" these data for PBR purposes makes eminent sense. Using available case records, client intake forms, client satisfaction questionnaires, records of previously conducted focus groups, computerized information systems and electronic records, etc., CDM is both grounded in practice, efficient and since it is generally retrospective does not interfere in any way with practice. Indeed, in most CDM studies, the practice that is being studied has already taken place.

CDM has been successfully employed by social workers and allied health practitioners in child welfare, family service, health and mental health settings throughout the world (Epstein *et al.*, in press; Plath and Gibbons, 2010; Joubert and Epstein, 2005; Peake, Epstein and Medeiros 2005; Epstein and Blumenfield, 2001). CDM has been used to document client needs, the adherence to and/or "fidelity" of "best practice" practice interventions and service outcomes. Sainz and Epstein (2001) have even explored how CDM studies can be used to more ethically approximate the cause–effect value of RCTs so that client randomization and the denial of service in control groups might be avoided in PBR.

Though ideally suited to PBR, CDM is not without its weaknesses and limitations. Since it relies on available data, CDM is only as good as the data that are available. Indeed the bane of CDM is missing data. So if you and other practitioners do not validly, reliably, accurately and fully record information concerning that which your study is intended to uncover, you are likely to come away from a data-mining effort empty handed. Still, Epstein (2010) has argued that just the process of conceptualizing the study and discovering what information isn't recorded can be highly informative and at the very least can improve future record keeping.

Since CDM is so compatible with PBR, once you have identified your study question, our advice is that you begin every PBR study by first asking what data are already available that might shed light on this question? Another approach is to begin with what data are already available and think about how these data might be used to answer one or more practice-relevant questions. When little is available and/or you have serious reasons to doubt its validity and reliability, then original data collection is the only option.

MIXED-METHOD STUDIES AND DATA COLLECTION

As you might expect mixed-method studies refer to studies that combine both qualitative and quantitative data collection and analysis (Creswell, 2009). Pushing the definition a bit further, Epstein *et al.* (in press), have added the use of available and original data to the mix. Thus, retrospective quantitative CDM studies based on available quantitative data can be enriched with prospective and original qualitative interview data.

So for example, Mirabito (2000) conducted her doctoral dissertation focusing on the "termination" phase in mental health counseling with adolescents particularly interested in why some clients end treatment precipitously and without warning. Since the quantitative CDM portion of the study raised more questions than it answered and presented findings that defied "practice wisdom" she followed up with original, follow-up interviews with clients who had ended treatment to find out why. The original qualitative data collection and analysis turned out to be especially helpful in explaining her unanticipated findings (Mirabito, 2000).

Alternatively, studies can begin with qualitative data and follow with a quantitative phase. Traditionally, academic researchers have suggested that mixed-method studies should "progress" from qualitative studies that conceptualize issues and generate hypotheses to quantitative studies that more rigorously "test" them. In this position, which is generally taken by post-positivists and RBP researchers, hypothesis-testing with quantitative data collection and analysis are the ultimate objective of research enquiry. While this approach to mixed-method research is certainly reasonable, it tends to "privilege" quantitative research at the expense of qualitative. Rubin (2008) counters this notion as misunderstanding EBP, contending that there are hierarchies of evidence depending on the practice question. He suggests that for some questions qualitative studies would be at the top of the evidence chain and RCTs at the bottom, while for others it may be the reverse. Our "methodologically pluralist" PBR position is intended to avoid such a pro-quantitative bias.

Those researchers who recognize the usefulness of following quantitative research with qualitative, emphasize the illustrative and explanatory uses of qualitative data collection and analysis. Mirabito's (2000) study cited above, does both. In her PBR doctoral dissertation, she began by conducting an initial series of original qualitative interviews in order to synthesize "grounded-theory" of precipitous termination derived from practitioners' "tacit knowledge" (Imre, 1985). She then tested this theory using quantitative CDM and when the data did not support the theory, she sought explanation with original qualitative data (Mirabito, 2000).

In her doctoral study of Filipino domestic workers' living conditions in New York City and return-migration intentions, Rajudaran (2010) was fortunate enough to have access to available quantitative and qualitative data from a membership survey and focus groups conducted in a voluntary association that advocates for these women. Here the qualitative portion of her study more richly described the working and living conditions of these women and explained why her quantitative findings did not yield what she anticipated based on prior research on other migrant groups. Similarly, Reeser and Epstein (1990) have suggested that a follow-up qualitative study of the meaning of the term "profession" be explored qualitatively as a follow-up to their original quantitative survey research on professionalization and social worker activism (Epstein, 2010).

In recent years, mixed-method studies have become somewhat fashionable among social work doctoral students and some academic researchers, the way qualitative research became a decade or so ago. There is now a *Journal of Mixed-Method Research*, research texts dedicated to this approach (Creswell, 2009) and doctoral courses teaching it. Consistent with our PBR position, while we support mixed-method studies we do not recommend them as ends-in-themselves. In other words, there needs to be a reason to be collecting both qualitative and quantitative data since multiple sources of data are likely to be more costly in worker time and effort. In addition, the more original data collection from clients, the more burdensome the study is likely to be.

Here as elsewhere, strategic compromise is required so that the desire for more data is balanced by a concern for cost and for clinical or programmatic intrusiveness.

SUMMARY OF KEY CONCEPTS

This chapter provided information regarding the key measurement concepts of reliability, validity, operationalization, and levels of measurement. We detailed the distinction between nominal, ordinal, interval and ratio levels of measurement. Quantitative data sources were explored, including the main characteristics of standardized scales, and ways to construct your own survey instrument. Consistent with the non-invasive principles of PBR we emphasized the potential to mine existing clinical data files or secondary databases. We also explored the potentially useful strategy of conducting a mixed-method PBR study.

Chapter 9

PBR sampling

Purpose

This chapter introduces the full array of sampling strategies available to you as a PBR researcher so you can make informed choices about the use of sampling in your study. Topics covered include the purposes of sampling, different sampling strategies, and the issue of sample size.

INTRODUCTION

Sampling is a research tool that both RBP and PBR researchers employ routinely. Simply stated, it involves studying a sub-set of units of analysis (e.g. individuals, case records, programs, etc.) and generalizing the findings to a larger population from which the sample was drawn. Strategies for doing so are especially useful to PBR researchers because they increase the efficiency and reduce the material costs and time involved in conducting practice research. Most importantly in PBR research, sampling reduces the potential burden on practitioners as well as on clients of doing or being involved in research.

Once you have refined your problem of interest, decided on the purpose of your study, selected a design, and developed a data-gathering strategy, then you are ready to consider who or what you want to study and ultimately what population you want to make a generalization about. Researchers refer to this as the universe about which you would like to make a statement. Of course, if you are studying a client population the ideal is to study the entire universe. This is true in RBP and in PBR alike. However, neither RBP nor PBR researchers always have the resources and time to study the entire population of clients, programs or community members about whom they'd like to either describe or make a causal statement. Practitioner-researchers (for whom research is not a primary role, and who are sensitive about the burdens research places upon both themselves and service recipients) find sampling strategies especially helpful in this regard. But, as with research designs, some "ideal" sampling strategies are more suited to RBP than they are to PBR. Here again a conflict exists between research rigor (for example, what strategy allows for the safest generalization?), its external validity, and the cost of implementation to both practitioners and study subjects.

This chapter explores a range of sampling strategies, some that lend themselves most easily to PBR, and some that fit less well but are favored by RBP researchers. However, as with design and data-gathering strategies, it is important as a practitioner-researcher that you understand the full array of sampling choices available, and then make sampling decisions that are most compatible with your practice priority, your study purpose and design. Here again a strategic compromise is likely to be called for.

The type of sampling strategy you choose, either probability or non-probability, will impact the extent to which you can generalize the findings of your research to different groups. It will also impact whether you can estimate the extent to which your generalization might be incorrect. This is important because whenever you sample, there is a probability – however small – that those sampling units not sampled will be quite different from those sampled. When they are, generalizations are incorrect.

This chapter identifies the differences between probability samples and non-probability samples, as well as the different sampling strategies that apply to each. For probability sampling we will explore simple random sampling, systematic random sampling, stratified random sampling, and cluster sampling. For non-probability sampling we will explore convenience sampling, purposive sampling, snowball sampling, and quota sampling. Having established the types of sampling strategies available we will discuss factors involved in choosing the right sampling strategy for your study. We will also consider the implications of your sampling strategy and sample size on the impact of your study findings, exploring the concepts of generalizability, and external validity. The chapter concludes with a discussion of how to determine sample size, and how to resolve sampling issues in PBR studies.

THE PURPOSE OF A SAMPLE

Your study sample refers to the people or cases that you are gathering data about or from. Your sampling strategy is how you select those people or cases for inclusion in your study. In principle, in any study the ideal would be to not sample at all but to study the entire universe of units of analysis. This ideal is achievable even in PBR studies when the universe is small and the possibility of surveying, interviewing, observing or analyzing case records is feasible, economical and relatively non-burdensome. So, when your study question applies to only a very small number of people or case records you may want to gather data from all of them (with their permission of course). This eliminates the worry about whether it is safe to generalize from your findings.

For example, if you are doing a needs study in which community leaders are going to be interviewed as "key informants", you would ideally identify all such individuals and interview them all. This would naturally require you to define what you mean by "community leader", locate them and invite them to participate in the study. If they all agreed then this would be called a universal sample. Likewise, if you were doing an after-only outcome survey of 40 previously abusive mothers who had received parenting training to prevent subsequent child abuse, you would want to survey all those who participated in the training sessions. However, even here the logic of sampling is valuable because in each instance it's quite possible (even probable) that not everyone will agree to be interviewed as in the first study, or complete and return your after-only questionnaire as in the second. In fact, many may not. So, as with studies in which sampling was intentionally employed, the differences between respondents and non-respondents would be of interest in making a generalization from the respondent population to the universe of community leaders or formerly abusive mothers, respectively. Hence even universal studies that involve small populations may require thinking and some kind of data collection about non-respondents.

In many PBR research efforts, however, the study question applies to a large number of people or cases and you simply don't have the time and resources to study all of them. Consequently, you will have to select some of those people to gather data from, and then apply your findings back to the larger group. Here, in addition to formal sampling logic, you may use to the same logic you might employ when you are cooking and you test whether or not your food is properly cooked. If you require a technical term for this, let's call it spaghetti logic.

So, for example, you use sampling *aka* spaghetti logic when you are cooking pasta, tasting one strand to test whether it is cooked to your liking, then you make a decision about all of the pasta based on that one test strand. To be even more certain you may test a second strand. In essence, you have taken a sample of the spaghetti and then applied what you learned to the whole pot. This is exactly what you do in research – you take a sample of the people or case records or programs or communities to which the research question applies and then make inferences from them to apply to the rest of the population of units of analysis. So, if you are thinking that studying your entire population of universe is not feasible, consider sampling. The following section explores different ways that you can select your sample, which are called sampling strategies. You can try some of them the next time you cook pasta!

TYPES OF SAMPLING

As indicated earlier, basically there are only two types of sampling – probability sampling and non-probability sampling. In probability sampling you can calculate each person's chance of being included in the sample and by implication the likelihood that the generalization drawn from the sample is valid. In order to employ probability sampling, you must know the size of the entire population to which the question applies, and how many units you have the resources to sample. Ideally, you would also know the distribution of key variables in the sample universe as well.

So, if you know that 100 people called your anti-bias hotline last month and you want to review 20 of the case records to see what the presenting issues were, then each case would have a known (20 out of 100 or 1 in 5) chance of being selected. From intake information on all 100, you might have information about gender, age, reason for call, etc. to which you can compare those in your sample to see how representative your sample is. Representativeness is a central objective of sampling and refers to the extent to which the distribution of key variables in the universe is mirrored in the sample. When that's true, it is safe to generalize findings from the sample to the universe. Thus, if our sample of 20 involved 50 percent men and 50 percent women but the universe of callers involved 25 percent men and 75 percent women, our sample would not be representative and generalizations about hotline "callers" would be suspect. If our study question concerned how men callers and women callers differed in their reasons for calling, this 50/50 distribution would be ideal. However, if our concern was primarily about the kinds of calls and requests for help that came in to the hotline in general, our sample would be problematic because men would be over-represented and women under-represented and that might have implications for the types of calls that came in.

Naturally, the larger the sample drawn, the higher the probability of achieving representativeness. Naturally as well, increasing the sample size adds to the costs and burden on the researcher and the respondent if original data are being collected. But sometimes the cost of increasing the sample size is small, relative to the advantages associated with greater confidence in the generalizability of the findings. This is particularly true in self-administered questionnaires and in using available data (e.g. case records) when data extraction is not labor-intensive (e.g. when only identifying information and simple, easily-identifiable intervention and outcome measures are used).

Even when you know little about the distribution of key variables in the universe, when you use a probability sample for your PBR study and the sample is large enough, the results that you get can be safely generalized. In that instance, you make an assumption that the things you found out about your sample also apply to the larger population. We call this the study's external validity, that is the extent to which the study findings are valid external to the people directly studied. So, in our relatively small example of 20 cases sampled from your anti-bias hotline to describe the presenting issues, if we knew that the sample was representative on gender and we determined that 45 percent of the calls were related to verbal abuse and violence while 55 percent of them were related to physical abuse and violence, from that we would safely assume similar proportions of presenting issues for the whole population of 100 cases. If we knew nothing about the gender distribution in the total sample of callers, we'd be a bit more cautious about generalizing the findings. But while we might think we knew the relationship between gender and presenting problem we still couldn't say anything about that in the total population, nor in the study population until we actually analyzed that relationship empirically in the study population.

Of the two basic types of sampling, probability sampling is the more rigorous from a research point of view and provides the safest inferences as well as a measure of how safe those inferences are. It's what we refer to as statistical significance which essentially tells you how safe it is to generalize from a sample to a total population. As you might expect, probability sampling is preferred by academic and RBP researchers for precisely those reasons. More will be said about this later in this chapter.

By contrast to the more rigorous probability sampling, in non-probability sampling it is not possible to estimate the person's, or case's or study unit's chances of being included in the sample because you don't know how big the population is that the sample is being drawn from. Likewise, you have no empirical data about the distribution of key variables in the universe. This is quite often the case in social work as we regularly deal with populations of an unknown size and unknown characteristics: for example, it is not possible to measure how many homeless people there are in Chicago, or how many people in Los Angeles were victims of domestic violence (since it is under-reported), nor do we necessarily know how many people might need our services. In these cases we do not know how big the potential pool of participants is and so we cannot calculate their chances of being included in the sample. And because we don't know what their gender or ethnic characteristics are, we cannot compare our ultimate sample with the universe so we can't make statistical inferences about how closely our sample represents our population, and we are not able to generalize the findings back to the population as a whole. Often however, given the information we have and don't have and the limited resources we have, non-probability sampling is the best we can do.

Hence, if you were practicing at AVP (New York City's Anti-Violence Project) where you know little about the universe of victims of violence since so many go unreported, but instead of wanting to describe the presenting issues of the callers to your hotline, you wanted to understand how the people that reached out to AVP compared with those who had experienced a bias crime but had not reached out to AVP, then to obtain a non-probability sample you may do outreach to groups for people who have experienced violence, to other social service agencies, or advertise through newspapers or via social networking sites. Using these techniques you may get a sample to ask your questions to, but in this case you would not be able to tell the size of the population that you are pulling your sample from, since you still do not know exactly how many people in New York City have experienced bias-related violence and are, therefore, potentially eligible for your study.

When you use a non-probability sampling strategy for your PBR study, you do not try to make inferences about how the findings apply to other people in the universe. Instead, you acknowledge that the results of the study only reflect the sample that you studied. While the findings can't be generalized beyond your immediate study sample, it still provides important practice and policy data related to your sample. This is often the case in exploratory quantitative research studies and in qualitative research where complex processes are studied in depth. In both instances, representativeness and generalizability are less important than gaining insight into a phenomenon that has not been previously studied at all, in the former, or in as great a depth as in the latter. Such a strategic compromise is made fairly frequently by RBP and PBR researchers alike.

Both probability and non-probability sampling techniques have a number of subtypes, which are important for the PBR researcher to know about. By knowing about these different sampling options, if sampling is required for your PBR study, you can decide which makes most sense for your study purpose, design and your available resources. Remember that the ideal is not to have to sample at all, but if sampling is required and you are doing a quantitative study then probability samples are preferred. If that is not possible or feasible or if you are doing a qualitative study, a non-probability is quite acceptable and sometimes even preferred.

PROBABILITY SAMPLING OPTIONS

Simple random sampling

This is the research equivalent of pulling numbers out of a hat, and can work well for PBR studies depending on the study context and the chosen design. What distinguishes a simple random sample from all other kinds of sampling types, is that each individual has an equal probability of being selected from the first selection to the last. Also, many statistical techniques that are employed in quantitative analysis are based on the assumption of simple random sampling. These data-analytic techniques tell us about the strength of relationships (i.e. effect size) as well as how safe it is for us to generalize from the sample to the universe. So sample size as well as how the sample is drawn are important considerations because they may rule out using our most powerful statistical techniques.

To draw a simple random sample you must begin with a complete listing of possible participants or units of analysis that are eligible for your study and assign a number to each from 1 to the end of the list. This also makes it possible to de-identify the individuals or cases by dropping ID numbers such as Social Security or Patient IDs that you wouldn't want in your data. A record of these and the new single number assigned should be kept in some safe place in case you need to match data from multiple sources (see Chapter 10 for more information about how to protect the confidentiality of data). However, once you have de-identified data then you can be sure that your analysis places no one's anonymity at risk.

Once you have a complete listing and case numbers assigned to each individual or case record, you can use a table of random numbers or a computer generated random numbers program to tell you which participants you should pull to put into the sample for your study until you reach your intended sample size (see Box 9.1 for an example).

In our anti-bias program example you wanted to draw a sample of 20 from the 100 cases. Once you have labelled all 100 cases you then select a method to draw the random sample. If you use a computer to generate your sample you would input the number of cases you have in the population (100) and the number of cases you would like in your sample (20), the computer would then generate a random list of 20 numbers between 1 and 100. (A number of statistical programs including Excel and SPSS or statistics websites like Stat Trek – http://stattrek.com/Tables/Random.aspx – will help you to draw random numbers.)

Once you have the random numbers selected, you match the cases in the database to the numbers in the sample, and then you either contact the people for inclusion in the study or pull the relevant case. Whatever the unit of analysis is the procedure is the same – assign each unit a number, select a random set of numbers and then include the corresponding unit in your study. The procedure is similar when using a hard copy of a table of random numbers rather than a computer program (see Box 9.1 for a description of drawing a random sample using a random numbers table). If you do not have a random numbers table or a computer at hand then you can simply put numbers into a hat (in this case 1–100) and pull 20 of them!

To use the random numbers table you take your sampling frame (the list of all potential participants) and assign each potential participant or case on the list a

BOX 9.1   DRAWING A RANDOM SAMPLE USING A
            RANDOM NUMBERS TABLE

A table of random numbers is usually formatted with several columns each containing a long list of 5, 6, or 7 digit numbers. Here is a 5-digit example:

03574	08651	75098	03403	65759	04571	03609	82901
12145	09675	19872	87934	23439	02745	09875	45329
75649	28390	84223	49783	56338	19394	64747	59092
39473	40987	49587	89549	58723	40895	72348	95349
85702	49834	29752	40389	57340	28953	40897	50482
92750	89247	54875	87205	78290	58485	74039	85702
49852	40578	20947	85049	87594	85724	98759	00875
82479	50894	78345	70985	78758	43275	78324	85702
93493	49045	32870	05894	72029	24857	23485	34834
70298	57098	47254	25874	28502	84735	08742	30863

number, then you take the random numbers table, close your eyes and place your finger anywhere on the table. Wherever your finger lands is your starting point on the list (this avoids any bias that might happen if you always started selecting your random numbers from the same place). In order to create as much variety as possible you decide whether you are going to read from left to right or right to left and whether you are going to read from top to bottom or bottom to top. Once you have decided, you read the number and include it in your sample if it falls within the range of numbers that you are looking for, so if you have the list from 1–100 and the first random number is 036, you would include it in the sample. But, if the number is 936, then you ignore that number and move onto the next number, since it falls beyond the scope of your sampling frame. Then you continue, including numbers that fall within the sampling frame and ignoring numbers that fall beyond the scope of your frame or that are a repeat of numbers that have already been included, until you have reached the 20 cases needed to fill your sample.

As we said earlier, in simple random sampling every case (or element) in the sampling frame (population) has an equal unbiased and known chance of being included in the sample. So for our example every member of the list has a 20 out of 100 (1 in 5) chance of being included in the sample – everyone's chances are known (we can calculate them), equal and unbiased (the same as everyone else's). This reduces the likelihood of sampling bias. We assume that the characteristics of the group are randomly distributed throughout the group and so will occur in the sample at similar rates as they occur in the population.

Systematic random sampling

This is also frequently used in PBR as it does not require a computer program or access to a random numbers table. It is relatively easy to implement and under most circumstances will produce a sample as varied and unbiased as a simple random sample. In systematic random sampling, cases are selected at a specific pre-set interval after a random starting point. So, for example, every 3rd or 5th or 10th case might be included in your study depending on the size of the sample you want and the size of the total population from which the sample is selected. The undefined interval between cases selected is referred to as k in statistical formulas. So, every k case is selected for inclusion in the sample depending on the size of the population and the size of the sample needed. Once you have chosen the appropriate interval then k is replaced in the formulas with the number that you have chosen (10 in our example).

To generate a systematic random sample you begin just as with simple random sampling, by making a list of all the possible cases to be included in the sample and assigning each case a number. Next, you select the size of your interval. To select the interval size you divide the total number of cases by the number you would like in your sample, your answer is your interval.

If we continue with the anti-bias program example and you have decided to use systematic random sampling, you would proceed by taking the caller population listing of 100 cases, and you want to take a sample of 20 of those cases, then you would divide the size of your population (100) by the size of the sample that you would like (20), to get an interval of 5 (100 ÷ 20 = 5), so you would take a random starting point from 1 to 5 and then take every 5th case from the entire list and include them in your study. As with simple random sampling, in systematic random sampling at the beginning every case (or element) has an equal and known chance of being included in the sample – in this case again it is 20 out of 100 or 1 in 5. However, once the first individual is selected, everyone else is determined. Still, we can generally assume that unless there is a bias in how the cases are ordered, there will be no bias in the sample. If we had a larger sampling frame and wanted to sample 100 out of 1000, we would proceed in exactly the same manner.

Systematic random sampling can work well with PBR studies, as it is possible to select case files from the filing cabinet by pulling each file that falls at the selected interval without having to make a list of all the file names or numbers first. If you use this method, make sure that all the files are in the cabinet before you begin, as if one worker has a number of his or her case files in the office, then his or her client's chances of inclusion in the study may be decreased. Another note of caution when using systematic random sampling is to be alert for any bias that may be evident in the way the population that you use to draw your sample from is listed. If your population list that you were going to draw your sample from was of sibling pairs and the oldest was always listed first, then any even numbered interval that you selected (e.g. 2, 4 or 6) would select only youngest siblings, and any odd numbered interval (e.g. 3, 5 or 7) would select only the oldest siblings.

Stratified random sampling

This form of sampling divides the population into groups or strata based on a specific characteristic that is central to the study purpose and then draws simple random or systematic random samples from each of the groups created. Stratified random sampling can be particularly useful when you want your sample to accurately reflect the proportional representation of certain groups within your population, for example, if you are studying MSW students and you want your sample to accurately reflect the proportion of first and second year students or students from different tracks in an MSW program.

Drawing a stratified random sample is done in two stages, first you stratify or divide the group based on one or more characteristic(s) and then you draw a random sample from the groups created. For example, if you were studying young people at your foster care agency and you wanted to ensure that you included children in kinship foster care and children in non-kinship foster care, then first you would create two sub-sets. The first stratum would include all the children in kinship foster care and the second would include all of the children not in kinship foster care. You would then draw a random sample from each pot – one representing the kinship foster care children and one representing the non-kinship foster care children. Every child (element) in each sub-set has an equal and known chance of being drawn from that pot (stratum).

In this more refined form of probability sampling, everyone in the population still has a known chance of being included in the sample because you can calculate each person's odds of being included. Note however that everyone in the population does not necessarily have an equal chance of being included in the sample unless you pull proportionately equivalent samples from each group. In this example, if there are 40 children in kinship foster care and you pull a random sample of 10 children, then each kinship foster child would have a 1 in 4 chance of being included in the sample. And, if there are 120 children in non-kinship foster care and you pull a random sample of 20 of them, then each non-kinship foster care child has a 1 in 6 chance of being included in the sample. Therefore, they have a known chance of being included in the sample (you know their odds) but not an equal chance, because the kinship children have a better chance of being included than the non-kinship children.

Quite often, in PBR studies there are times when you want to "over-sample" one group to give you a chance to really learn about them for practice purposes. So, if we return to our anti-bias program (ABP) research for example, perhaps of those 100 calls that come in to the hotline, 12 were from people identifying as transgender or gender queer, while 62 callers were male identified and 26 were female identified. In that case you may want to ensure that some or even all of the transgender/gender queer cases are included in your analysis, so you may stratify the cases by gender and then select a sample from each stratum. Perhaps you chose to select 12 cases from each stratum, then the transgender cases have a greater chance of being selected (12/12) than those that identified as female (12/26) and they would both have a greater chance of being included in the sample than those identified as male (12/62).

Sometimes our preference is to draw the samples in such a way that they match the proportions in the larger population. This is what we would call proportionate, stratified random sampling. In studies where we over-sample some and under-sample others, we call it disproportionate, stratified random sampling. In the ABP study, we would choose the former sampling strategy to maximize the descriptive similarity between our sample and the agency population on gender. On the other hand, if we were most interested in comparing female and male callers, we would use a disproportionate sampling strategy, over-sampling the men and under-sampling the women. All would depend on our study purpose.

Cluster random sampling

Also referred to as multi-level or multi-stage sampling, cluster random sampling draws random samples in stages from a series of naturally occurring groups (clusters). Cluster random sampling is most often used when the size or spread of the population being studied is so large that it is not feasible to draw a simple or systematic random sample without first partializing the population into smaller more manageable units (see Box 9.2 insert for a specific example). Though rarely used in small PBR studies, cluster random sampling might be useful in larger, policy-oriented surveys, for example, if you wanted to look at cases across the health care system or the child welfare system in a particular city or state, or if your agency was part of a large network of agencies and you wanted to draw a sample of clients from across the whole spectrum.

As an example, if you were using cluster random sampling in a study of customer satisfaction of social work services across a large network of hospitals, you would first divide the country into states where there are hospitals from the network, and take a random sample of those states. Then you would draw a random sample of hospitals from those states. You would next draw a random sample of units from those hospitals, before finally drawing a random sample of patients from those units. In this way you have drawn a random sample of patients across the hospital network, without having had to create a list of every single patient in every single hospital.

All of the methods discussed above are probability samples and are applied when you know the parameters of the universe or total population that you want to study. However, very often in PBR you do not have a detailed enumeration of those who fall into your population of interest.

In these cases we use non-probability sampling methods in which individuals do not have an equal or known chance of being included in the sample. And, from which any conclusions drawn can only be applied to the participants being studied, the results cannot be statistically generalized to the larger population of interest. However, non-probability samples do generate valuable findings and the inability to use probability sampling should not deter you from conducting research when sampling is required. This is especially true when the PBR study proposed is exploratory and will lead to subsequent, more rigorous research.

NON-PROBABILITY SAMPLING OPTIONS

Convenience/accidental sampling

This form of sampling is exactly as it sounds, convenient and unsystematic. (It is often confused, however, with random sampling which sounds "accidental" and "convenient" but it is neither.) In convenience sampling, you access people who are available

BOX 9.2   DRAWING A CLUSTER RANDOM SAMPLE OF INDIVIDUALS IN THE UNITED STATES

To use cluster sampling to draw a random sample of individuals in the United States you would start with a map of the US and divide it into the 50 states. You would then draw a random sample of those states (say 10 states). You would divide that pot into counties (say 100 counties), and from those counties you would draw a random sample of say 25. You would then divide those 25 counties into street blocks (say 5000 blocks) and draw a random sample of 250 blocks. You would then divide those 250 blocks into households (say 3000 households) and then draw a sample of 300 households. You would then divide the households into individuals (say 1200) and you would draw a random sample of 400. This process would give you a random sample of 400 citizens of the United States.

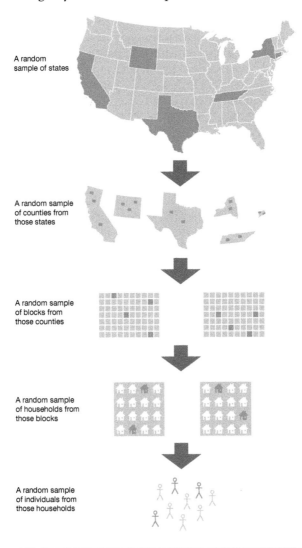

A random sample of states

A random sample of counties from those states

A random sample of blocks from those counties

A random sample of households from those blocks

A random sample of individuals from those households

to you for some reason; perhaps they come to your agency for services, attend your program, are residents in your community, belong to an organization that you know, or simply answer the telephone when you call.

For example, you may be interested in understanding the social service needs of individuals within the neighbourhood community where your agency is located. To do this, you decide to interview people, at a community street fair that is held each June. The sample of individuals that you draw is a convenience or accidental sample comprised entirely of people who happened to attend the festival and were willing to be interviewed. You know nothing about how they differ from those who do not attend the festival, nor do you know anything about those who attend but refuse to be interviewed.

Still, the interviews can be very helpful to you as you begin to plan social services for that particular neighbourhood. Perhaps these are the people who would be most likely to reach out to the agency? Perhaps not? Certainly, your findings cannot be said to be in some statistical sense, representative of the service needs of the community as a whole, but rather only of those individuals who completed the interview. Nonetheless, the results give you an idea of what some people in the neighbourhood think and this is better than total speculation. At the same time we recognize that those who attended this community event did not include people who were not well enough to leave the house that day. These individuals may be most in need of particular types of services, perhaps some in-home services for example. Perhaps the street festival is more appealing to some cultural groups rather than to others, or to some age groups rather than to others, or perhaps it draws more families? In this way, it is not possible to know the representativeness of the sample. But, you do know the needs identified by the people you did talk to. And, knowing what you don't know, you can follow up with some kind of door-to-door or telephone survey in the future.

When interpreting and reporting the results from a convenience sample it is important to be clear that they are reflective only of your sample and may not be reflective of the larger group. Some have argued that convenience samples can provide misleading information and may be even worse than having no sample at all (Neuman, 2007, for example). We disagree however. In PBR, if sampling is necessary, a convenience sample may be the best available sample and we would argue that it is useful as long as there is clarity about the limits to whom the findings apply and attempts are made to anticipate and to gather data from all relevant groups, so that as many voices as possible are included in your sample.

Snowball sampling

Snowball sampling is a particular type of convenience sampling that can be used when you are trying to study a population or group that is particularly hard to identify or gain access to. This is often the case when you are trying to study stigmatized populations, stigmatized behaviors, or hard to reach populations such as intravenous drug users, survivors of domestic violence, commercial sex workers, LGBT individuals, or homeless youth.

In snowball sampling, you start with a few people who you know and who meet the criteria of your study, then you ask them to recommend other people who would also be appropriate. From there, you ask those individuals to recommend others, and so on until you have either exhausted all of your possible leads or you have achieved your sample size. In snowball sampling it is important to develop the trust of your participants with relevant and non-exploitive research, so that your participants will recommend your study to their friends. Snowball sampling is not unlike the outreach that social workers do when they are trying to encourage hard-to-reach groups to access services and thus it is quite compatible with PBR.

Quota sampling

This is the non-probability equivalent of stratified random sampling, and is used when you are seeking to approximate proportionate representation of certain groups within your sample or disproportionate distribution where comparisons between sub-groups are sought. Quota sampling only makes sense, however, when you can roughly approximate the proportion of key characteristics in your study population. Perhaps at the street fair you tried to reach different ethnic groups in the same proportions as reside within the community. So, based on census data, if the street fair was in a neighborhood like East Harlem in New York City, where approximately 52 percent of the residents are Latino and 36 percent are African-American (United States Census Bureau, 2000) and you knew that Latinos were moving in since the last census, you might set quotas of 60 percent of Latinos, 35 percent of African-Americans and 5 percent others. Once you've met any of the quotas, you would stop approaching attendees who appeared to be from that group or who self-identified as such.

As with stratified random sampling you fill your sample trying to achieve particular rates of inclusion, but for quota sampling you do not randomly select them for inclusion – you select whoever is available to you. In other words, it's a convenience sample with pre-designated quotas. Despite your efforts to make your sample representative of the population, it is not a probability sample so the results still apply only to the sample of the study. Moreover, it should be clear that the prevailing advantage of randomized sampling procedures is that they maximize the likelihood of representation for variables that you know about and think are relevant to your study as well as variables that you haven't even thought about. That's why random assignment is employed in RCTs and why almost any probability sample is better than a non-probability sample. Arguably however, the one exception is purposive sampling.

Purposive sampling

Purposive sampling is a very specific type of convenience sampling often used in qualitative research. It involves actively seeking subjects that you think will have the specific combinations of characteristics that are relevant to your study. For this reason, purposive sampling is sometimes called theoretical sampling.

Thus, if you are interested in how a particular housing policy emerged, you would seek to interview legislative officials and lobbyists who were involved in the legislative process and you would want to be sure that you included those of each political party who voted for or against the legislation. Hence, your sampling frame would include both Republicans and Democrats who were for or against the legislation, assuming that all four types existed. Here, if the Democrats were the main supporters of the legislation, you might be particularly interested in Democrats who voted against it and Republicans who voted for it. These interviews may provide more insight into the emergence of the legislation than interviews with those more numerous legislators who voted along party lines.

Likewise, if you were wondering how well the service hours and services of your agency meets the needs of those families served by your agency with small children, then you would purposefully seek out agency clients with small children who were employed, as well as those who were unemployed. In addition, you might sample families in which grandmothers were major providers of childcare for their grandchildren. What makes purposive sampling ideal in qualitative research is that various theoretically relevant combinations of factors can be hand-selected whereas reliance on the probability of them appearing in your sample might be slim.

Purposive sampling is used very often with PBR qualitative studies where you reach out to people for interviews and focus groups which you think will have valuable information related to your question. Just as you would when you are creating a community advisory board, you try to create a sample that comprises a variety of perspectives. It is important to be aware of the potential for the sample to be biased by available voices that represent the dominant norm and to take steps to include a range of diverse voices wherever possible.

SAMPLE SIZE

In probability samples it is possible to calculate the size of the sample that you will need in order to know how confident you can be about your results. The goal is to study a practically feasible number of participants while minimizing sampling error. Sampling error refers to the difference between the responses of the total population and the answers of your sample. The bigger your study sample, the better the chance that it accurately reflects the group that you are sampling from (population), because a greater proportion of the population is included. The more closely the participants' scores match those of the total population, the smaller the sampling error.

Some samples that you draw will match the universe extremely well, some will deviate in one direction or another. Some will deviate a little and some will deviate a lot. The higher the proportion of the characteristic in the total population the more likely it is to show up in your sample. But that's only a probability and sometimes by chance alone our samples are widely skewed. However, achieving a large sampling ratio may not be feasible.

So, in our example of 100 cases from the anti-bias program, if you review the presenting issue for 90 out of 100 cases it will be very time-consuming but you will get responses that are a very close approximation to all 100 cases in the population. And there still may be 1 or 2 very unusual cases that you've missed. Alternatively, if you take only 20 cases then it will be much quicker, cheaper and less labor-intensive, but the findings are less likely to accurately reflect the full range of issues presented.

The law of diminishing returns applies, because the increase in sample size is not proportionate to the increase in accuracy. (There are tables that show the reduction in sampling error by sample size – see for example Craft, 1990, p.111, Table 8.1, or Anastas, 1999, p.280, Table 10.1, Rubin and Babbie, 1993, p.234, Table 8.1.) In this way deciding on the sample size for your random sample involves a "trade off between precision and feasibility" (Anastas, 1999, p.280). In addition to the size of the sample, sampling error is affected by how alike or how varied your study population is, which is called the homogeneity of your sample. If the population that you are drawing from is very similar (homogeneous) then you do not need as large a sample as when they are very different (heterogeneous).

In order to calculate the sample size needed you have to determine three things: the confidence level that you are applying, the confidence interval that you are willing to tolerate, and the size of the population. The confidence level of the study refers to the degree of certainty that you want to have that your sample's responses are reflective of their population. The three commonly used confidence levels are 99 percent, 95 percent and 90 percent depending upon your purpose of the study. If your study is exploratory then a 90 percent confidence level may be appropriate. However, if you are testing a new intervention for suicidality, then you'd want a very high degree of precision in your findings and so may apply a 99 percent confidence level. The most common confidence level in social science is the 95 percent confidence level, in which you are 95 percent sure that your sample's answers reflect the answers of the entire population within the confidence interval.

The confidence interval is most recognizable from Gallup and other TV and news polls. It is the range that you are willing to be "off" from the actual responses of the population that you are studying, and it is expressed as a + or – figure. So, when discussing the President's approval rating, a reporter may state that 48 percent of Americans approve of how the President is doing his job +/– 5 percent. In this case we would be sure that the accurate approval of the President for his job performance from the whole population is within the 43–53 percent range.

Once you have your confidence level and confidence interval determined, and you know the size of your population, then you can calculate the sample size that you need to meet these parameters. There are useful websites such as www.researchinfo. com/docs/calculators/samplesize.cfm which can help you. As an example, if you have set your confidence level at 95 percent , and you want a confidence interval of 5, and you have a population of 100, then you would need to draw 80 cases. However, if you tightened your confidence level to 99 percent and you want a confidence interval of 5, and you have a population of 100, then you would need to draw a sample of 87.

Moreover, there are statistical procedures for determining the relationship between sample size necessary given the level of causal certainty desired in RCTs and other hypothesis-testing studies being planned. These are especially useful in RBP studies and they are required in many grant applications. This desired degree of predictability between independent and dependent variables is referred to as the effect size. In practice research, it refers to how much variation in the outcome is accounted for by the intervention alone.

A statistical procedure called power analysis tells us what sample size is necessary for us to test cause–effect hypotheses with a desired degree of confidence. For our purposes, it is sufficient for you to know that this statistical technique exists, is generally required in research grants to justify the projected sample size and the possibility of sample attrition (i.e. people dropping out of the study over time). For a power analysis, you may need a statistical consultant, however in PBR as well as in many RBP studies sample size is usually more a matter of resources in time and money as well as issues of access than of anything else.

DECIDING ON A SAMPLING STRATEGY

As we have discussed, in deciding on a sampling strategy the criteria most often cited involve some compromise between precision – how closely your sample matches the characteristics of your whole population – and feasibility including the time, cost, and access you have. In PBR, however, a fourth and crucial feasibility factor emerges as perhaps the most salient – what makes the most practice sense? What is the best way to obtain a useable sample without disturbing, interrupting, or delaying service more than minimally?

The concept of strategic compromise is important again in sampling to determine the most representative sampling strategy possible while "normal" practice protocols are maintained. Does it make the most sense to gather data from participants prospectively as they join a particular treatment program, since new members are joining sufficiently frequently to make that seem viable? Or, since the client base is fairly stable, does it make more sense to sample all current clients, perhaps using random sampling? Or if the program has been running a long time and the particular type of client you are trying to access doesn't receive services in large numbers at any one time, then does it make more sense for you to draw a sample retrospectively from the case records of clients that fit the study criteria and were previously serviced by the program? These are practical and practice-relevant aspects of the sampling decision that weigh more heavily in PBR than they do in RBP.

If you choose to use retrospective data review to conduct a data-mining study (see Epstein, 2010), then it is important to be thoughtful about the timeframe that you designate to collect cases from. Be sure to take into account any major personnel, administration, program or policy changes that may have occurred in the interim, and carefully decide whether to draw a sample to include cases throughout or whether to limit data to a "window" before or after a particular change.

Two other factors that feature in PBR sampling decisions are the intent of your study, and your method of analysis. When considering the intent you ask what is the purpose of the study and how accurate do you need to be? If your study is exploratory and you are just beginning to look at an issue, or develop a sense of the relevant practice concept then a small convenience sample may make the most sense. On the other hand, probability sampling or not sampling at all but using the universe should be considered in studies that purport to describe certain characteristics of the group in precise ways.

Similarly, when considering your method of analysis, whether your study is quantitative or qualitative may affect the size of your sample. Some statistical calculations require a minimum number of cases in order for their formulas to function, for example in a chi-square test there is an assumption that simple random sampling is employed and that there will be a minimum of 5 subjects in each category of every table that is presented (see Chapter 12 for a discussion of chi-square). If you are worried about meeting statistical assumptions then you can apply a formula developed by Galtung (1967) to determine sample size ($rn \times 20$ = sample size, where r is the number of values in each variable, and n refers to the number of variables). Instead, some researchers use an approximation of 30 subjects as their baseline while others use 100 (Monette, Sullivan and DeJong, 1994). However, as indicated earlier, in PBR practice considerations always supersede statistical considerations.

DESCRIBING THE SAMPLE

By their very nature PBR studies are reflective of the practice context in which they are conducted and the populations on whom their results are based. So, when communicating about your study to others it is important to give a full description of your sample and how it was drawn including the extent to which it varies on demographic characteristics that might be relevant to the interpretation of your findings by others, like gender, age, race, ethnicity, socio-economic status, education level, sexual orientation, and marital status. You should also clearly describe the extent that the sample does or does not mirror the larger population. Obviously, in providing a thorough description you should be sure to honor human subjects protection protocols and provide no identifying individual, group, or organization information unless you have specific permission to do so (this will be discussed in greater detail in the next chapter). Finally, if a sizable number of individuals refuse to participate or fail to complete the study protocol, you should make every effort to describe the differences between those whose needs, knowledge, attitudes and/or behaviors are represented in the study data and those whose are not.

SUMMARY OF KEY CONCEPTS

This chapter offered reasons for sampling in PBR studies and highlighted the differences between probability and non-probability sampling strategies. While PBR often relies on non-probability sampling, specific strategies of both probability and non-probability can be adapted to PBR study purposes. Illustrations of each were provided. Key concepts covered included an exploration of sampling error, confidence intervals, confidence levels, generalizability and external validity. However, the importance of prioritizing practice protocols over research ideals was again offered as a central PBR principle.

Chapter 10

Research ethics and protection of human subjects in PBR

Purpose

Whenever human beings (and for that matter all sentient animals) are involved in research, ethical issues arise. Whether the involvement is active (e.g., participating in a focus group) or passive (e.g., having case records "mined" for data), every researcher must give serious attention to whether even the best intentioned research activity might do harm to those involved. This is most obvious in medical and pharmaceutical research but it applies as well to social work research. And, it matters little whether the person doing the research is a "famous" research professor or a social work student conducting a small-scale study for that professor's research course assignment. In pursuing knowledge, the watchwords for both are do no harm.

This chapter discusses the historical roots of our concern for the "protection" of those involved in our research studies. With regard to research more generally, we discuss in detail two central ethical principles for conducting research with human subjects – fully informed consent and confidentiality. More specifically, in the context of PBR, we debate the ethics of conducting randomized controlled trials (RCTs) from a social work perspective. We end with a note about institutional review boards (aka ethics committees, human subjects committees, etc.) and their important role in the protection of study participants.

INTRODUCTION

As a social worker, wherever you are and whatever your form of practice, you are bound by a code of ethics that outlines the expectations for your professional conduct (see, for example the NASW code in the US, the AASW code in Australia, the BASW code in Britain, the CASW code in Canada, and the IFSW code throughout the world). These ethical codes provide not only guidance for your actions but also standards against which your practice can be judged.

Similar to professional codes of ethics, research ethics provide guidelines for morally appropriate behavior when conducting research. The purpose of research ethics and the institutional review boards, or human subjects committees, that interpret and enforce them is to protect the "subjects" (we prefer the term participants) who are involved in research studies, especially those who are vulnerable or over whom the researcher may be seen to hold power, such as young children, people in institutions, or individuals with learning disabilities. In some settings, these committees also view their function as assuring the quality of the research conducted. In research centers attached to teaching hospitals, these functions may be separated into two separate committees, human subjects committees and scientific standards committees. Of course this raises the possibility of conflicts between human subject protection and knowledge generation. Indeed, sometimes the two are incompatible. In PBR, when this happens, to the extent possible, we clearly align ourselves with our best understanding of the interests of service recipients rather than "gold standard" views of science.

In this chapter we outline the historical antecedents of IRBs, we discuss the role of IRBs, and we draw attention to particular ethical pitfalls that practitioner-researchers should avoid in order to:

1   ensure fully informed consent;
2   ensure inclusive language;
3   maintain confidentiality;
4   once data are collected, to promote secure information management.

In discussing the foregoing ethical principles, we are eager that you don't view research ethics and the IRBs that oversee and enforce them as a barrier to your conducting PBR, but rather as another aspect of mindful, reflective and respectful practice, something for which, as a social worker, you are very well prepared and something that PBR promotes.

SO WHAT ARE ETHICS ANYWAY?

Before we begin our discussion about conducting ethical PBR studies, we need to address the question "what exactly are ethics?" This inevitably leads to a discussion about values upon which ethics stand. Values are those things that are deemed to be "right" or "good". Ironically, it is very hard to come up with a definition of values that doesn't include the word value or valuable in it – for example, Dolgoff and Skolnick (1992) define values as something "intrinsically valuable or desirable" to a society (p.100). In other words (well almost), values represent preferences that can guide our actions. Following from this, ethics are how we act on those values – they represent our values in action.

There is always an underlying set of values that frames ethical guidelines. In the US the National Association of Social Workers (NASW) describes the purpose of codes of ethics as to "set forth values, ethical principles, and ethical standards to which professionals aspire and by which their actions can be judged" (NASW, 2008, p.4). Accordingly, the NASW code of ethics outlines six underlying values that serve as the foundation for the code of ethics, namely service, social justice, dignity and worth of the person, importance of human relationships, integrity, and competence (NASW, 2008). The code of ethics outlines ways in which practitioners should act on those values as professional social workers. As a practitioner-researcher you have to respond to and integrate two sets of ethical guidelines: practice ethics and research ethics.

While you are probably already very familiar with the social work practice half of the equation, the rest of this chapter focuses on the research part. We start in the following section by discussing some significant events in the history of social research that led to the development of research ethics and mechanisms for their enforcement. Sadly, these events do not reflect very positively on the research enterprise. However, the codification of research ethics demonstrates how researchers are committed to not repeating these moral lapses of their predecessors.

ESTABLISHING A HISTORICAL IMPERATIVE FOR PROTECTION OF HUMAN SUBJECTS

Our mindfulness about the people we study as part of research today stems from the egregious actions of others in the past. The first code of research ethics was the Nuremberg Code, established in 1949 as a result of the revelation during the Nuremberg trials of atrocities that occurred in the name of "medical research" within Nazi concentration camps.

The code set out 10 key guidelines for future research including voluntary consent and avoiding unnecessary risks to the human subjects of the research. However, despite the existence of the Nuremberg code, evidence of subsequent unethical studies within the USA led to federal research guidelines as part of a report by the Surgeon General in 1966 (Kitchener and Kitchener, 2009). In 1974, the National Research Act established institutional review boards and also the National Commission for the Protection of Human Subjects in Biomedical and Behavioral Research. The National Commission was formed to create a set of guiding principles for researchers, and their work resulted in the Belmont Report (1978). The principles of the Belmont Report, respect for persons, beneficence, and justice build on those from the Nuremberg code and are the foundation for the research ethics upheld in the USA today (see Box 10.1 for key dates in the history of social science research ethics).

Violations of these three principles were evident in some of the controversial research studies that led to the creation of these protections. For example, deception that caused significant psychological harm was central in Milgram's (1974) infamous obedience study where participants were instructed to administer increasingly strong pseudo "electric shocks" to other people that they did not know were actors hired by the researcher. The shocks were not real, but as the shocks were given, the actors shrieked and writhed in pain. Many of the study participants continued to administer what they believed to be increasingly strong and even potentially fatal "shocks" simply because they were told to do so by an authority figure.

Although Milgram's (1974) intention was to shed light on our propensity to be compliant in response to authority figures, he did so by inflicting extreme psychological harm on study participants who found themselves overriding their own ethical concerns while administering what they believed to be significant harm on other persons – all actors of course. Despite his higher purpose, Milgram's study called into question the human risks versus the knowledge benefits of the study and thus the notion of beneficence. In addition, it was responsible for the creation of informed consent procedures that reinforced the principle of respect for subjects recruited for research purposes.

Another research study that led to the creation of the commission was a study that lasted for 40 years but failed to provide fully informed consent and proper treatment to hundreds of African-American men infected with syphilis. What has become known today as the notorious Tuskegee syphilis study began in 1932 and was only brought to a halt in the 1970s (Jones, 1993). Study subjects were never told that they had syphilis, but were provided with free medical exams, free meals during their exams, experimental doses of penicillin and free burial in exchange for their participation. In 1997, President Clinton offered a public apology and a court ruling awarded financial compensation to the study survivors and their families, but not before many lost their lives and many wives and children had been unknowingly infected.

A third study often cited as part of the impetus for tighter oversight in research practices involved deception, invasion of privacy and lack of informed consent. In his studies of homosexual encounters in public restrooms termed the "tearoom trade", Laud Humphreys (1970) used a two-part system to gather his research data. Intending to understand more about those who participated in these same-sex (illegal) encounters, and whether they otherwise represented themselves as heterosexual, Humphreys himself acted as an observer and a "lookout" for those engaging in sexual acts. He then recorded the license plate numbers of the men he had observed and using his academic researcher bona fides was allowed to access motor vehicle records, names and addresses. Finally, he made follow-up house calls requesting their participation in an interview through which he gathered background and demographic information about these men – several of whom were married with children.

By doing this, Humphreys violated their privacy in multiple ways. Clearly, study "participants" were not in control of access to their identities or other personal information. While the men did formally consent to participate in the interview part of the study, they may have chosen not to had they been informed about the actual purpose of the research, and they were not given a choice whether to participate in the observation phase. Although the excesses of this study provoked additional human subjects protections some years later, it is not insignificant that at the time of its publication it won an award from the academically prestigious Society for the Study of Social Problems. Fortunately, since then the value placed on academic knowledge generation and the rights of research subjects has found a better balance.

Reflecting back on these morally objectionable events in research history, it is important to note that both the Nuremberg trials and the Tuskegee study involved the exploitation of minority groups, whereas Humphreys' involved a stigmatized group. Those given to conspiracy theories about academic research have credible evidence on which to stake their claim. As shameful as these examples were, they eventually led to corrective structures and principles whereby social research could continue but not at the expense of the human subjects participating in these studies.

A lesson for practitioner-researchers like yourselves is that as you develop your sampling and recruitment strategies for PBR studies you should remain mindful of the negative experiences that some have had in the past with "research". Make efforts to be thoughtful and fully informative in the language that you use, and dedicate time to ensuring your participants are comfortable with their involvement in your study and that you are purposeful in your attention to the diversity of your sample. It is also painfully ironic that the Tuskegee study used a number of best practices for culturally competent and ethnically sensitive methods to recruit participants to their study that are still valid today. The following section focuses on how you can protect the participants in your PBR studies.

KEY AREAS OF PROTECTION IN PBR

Now that we have noted a few of the most egregiously unethical episodes in the history of social research, let's focus on the positive principles of human subjects protection that emerged in response. Tutty, Rothery, and Grinnell (1996) identified three primary ethical concerns that apply to all social research studies involving human subjects. These are informed consent, confidentiality and management of information. The following section considers these three concerns specifically as they relate to PBR studies.

BOX 10.1   RESEARCH ETHICS: KEY DATES

1945   Nuremberg trials begin
1949   Nuremberg Code
1966   NIH Office of Protection of Research Risks (OPRR) created
1970   Humphreys' Tearoom Trade Study published
1972   Tuskegee Syphilis Study protocol revealed (study began in 1932)
1973   Congressional hearings on the Tuskegee Syphilis Study
1974   Milgram's Obedience Study book published (study began in 1961)
1974   National Research Act (creation of Institutional Review Boards)
1976   Federal Guidelines for Research in Surgeon General's Report
1978   National Commission for the Protection of Human Subjects in Biomedical and Behavioral Research created the Belmont Report
2000   OPRR made part of HHS and renamed Office of Human Research Protections (OHRP)
2002   Certificates of Confidentiality were created by the Public Health Services Act through the National Institute of Health

---

Generating fully informed consent

Since concerns about research as well as litigation have become intertwined with social work practice in recent years, many social work and allied health settings routinely ask consumers, clients or patients to sign consent forms of one kind or another at the beginning of the intake and assessment process. Obviously, the reason for this is to protect the agency and practitioners as well as service recipients.

The forms generally cover key issues for agency liability and outline consent for treatment. In some agencies this is also an opportunity for a blanket statement about the use of information gathered for program evaluation and other research purposes. When possible, in the spirit of fully informed consent we recommend adding your own study specific research consent procedures at the time you conduct your study, to any blanket statement that may already exist within your agency. Our reason for this position is that quite often the blanket consent is administered just as service is beginning, at a time when clients are especially vulnerable and perhaps eager to "get started". Clients may feel that they have to agree and sign any and all forms presented in order to make it to the next step of the process, i.e. actually receiving services. Ideally, we recommend engaging in an active consent process with your clients in relation to your specific PBR study (when applicable), and allowing participants to be very specific about the activities and uses of information to which they are consenting.

For example, perhaps they are consenting to an interview but not to being audio- or videotaped. Perhaps they are agreeing to the information being used to help the agency in their program planning but don't want it included in academic articles. Often you can create check boxes on the consent form so that individuals can designate the level of participation with which they are comfortable. We also urge you to make it very clear that their research consent signature is not required in order for them to receive services.

Box 10.2 outlines some of the key features of an informed consent procedure that you should follow when conducting your PBR study. Your agency's or institution's IRB may have additional guidelines that you will be required to follow.

The first responsibility of the informed consent process is to inform a potential participant of what is involved in the study. You are obliged to inform them about the following:

1   the purpose of your study;
2   the activities involved in your study;
3   how your findings may be used;
4   any potential risks or harms associated with participation;
5   any potential benefits or compensation for their participation.

Although we try as much as possible to fully achieve these principles, it is truly impossible for clients to give fully informed consent until they have seen all of the questions or been exposed to all of the "experimental conditions" (e.g. treatment interventions) involved in the study. Hence agreeing to participate in a program evaluation at intake is not the same as the experience of receiving treatment and complying with a post-treatment follow-up interview. However, current convention allows potential service recipients consumers to consent in theory and then stop participation at any point if they are no longer comfortable with their involvement.

Once the participant has been fully informed in relation to the study's purpose and procedures you can then secure consent or agreement to participate. Consent may be in the form of a signature for confidential studies or it may be implied in anonymous studies. For example, a statement before questions on an anonymous questionnaire would note that by completing the questions they are implying their consent to participate in your study. In the case of minors or others who have decision-making guardians parental or guardian consent should be established. For minors who are mature enough a separate procedure should be established to secure their assent to participate. (What constitutes "mature enough" is left to the researcher's discretion.) Here again, in the interest of preserving the client's rights, it is important that you clearly establish that parental consent does not obligate the young person to provide assent, just as assent does not ensure parental consent – they should be seen as two discrete processes both required in order to secure participation.

Given that in PBR studies a number of study participants may also be your clients or clients of your agency, there is a particular need to ensure that there is no coercion in the consent process, since there is always a danger that clients will be so eager to please you or seek your approval that they feel like they can't refuse.

Clearing your procedures with your agency's IRB or Human Subjects Research Committee or its equivalent will help to ensure that you are not unduly influencing your clients' consent decision. Anonymous participation, where the identity of participants is not known by anyone and is not traceable (e.g. by email address) is an ideal way to protect against inadvertent coercion, but not all studies lend themselves to an anonymous design. Where anonymity is not feasible then having other social workers or administrators conduct the outreach and recruitment, with no one directly engaging their own clients, can be helpful.

Before we move on from our discussion of informed consent it is important to say a few words about vulnerable populations for whom specific guidelines exist. Vulnerable populations include anyone under 18, individuals with physical or mental disabilities, pregnant women, and prisoners. You can imagine that some of these populations may not be equipped to make independent decisions or may feel as though they do not have sufficient autonomy to refuse to participate in a research study that someone with greater authority is asking them to participate in. Or they might fear that non-participation will expose them to negative consequences.

Imagine, for example, prisoners being asked to participate in a research study and feeling as though not doing so might be used as evidence of non-compliance, and thus jeopardizing their chances of parole. IRBs pay special attention to studies involving vulnerable populations and require that all research proposals are discussed before a full committee, with a person with experience with the vulnerable population (e.g. a prisoner or prisoner representative) present when applicable.

Many PBR studies inevitably involve vulnerable populations. Our purpose in emphasizing these issues is not to dissuade you from conducting research but rather to ensure that you engage these populations mindfully, sensitively and review your procedures to ensure that you are following sound informed consent protocols (see Box 10.2). And while our ultimate purpose is to seamlessly integrate practice and research, there are times in PBR studies when the lines between the two are blurred. By emphasizing ethical principles our intent is to assure that study participants' rights are not violated or taken for granted.

BOX 10.2 ELEMENTS OF INFORMED CONSENT

- A statement of purpose
- An explanation of how the participant came to be selected for inclusion
- Disclosure of who else is being asked to participate
- Duration of their expected participation
- Procedures to be followed during the study
- Extent that protocols are already established or new
- Description of potential risks
- Description of potential benefits
- Information related to other potentially helpful treatments that are currently available
- Extent that participation is anonymous or confidential and any limits to those
- Compensation if any to be provided
- Contact information in case they have further questions
- A clear statement regarding the voluntary nature of participation
- A clear statement that choosing whether or not to participate will not impact receipt of services
- A statement that the participant is free to stop participation at any point

---

Confidentiality and privacy

Confidentiality is a central tenet of all social work practice, and consequently is a concept with which we are sure you are familiar. Maintaining confidentiality of the information gathered during your PBR study is as central to the integrity of the research process as it is to the social work process. Just as in practice, in research confidentiality is maintained through discreet communications that do not identify the project; arranging study related interactions in private locations when appropriate; limiting access to information to those directly related to the study and who have direct permission; keeping all documentation secure; and, not revealing participants' identities in study findings or reports (e.g. providing aggregate rather than individual data when appropriate).

Given the nature of social work practice and the client populations with which you work, it is likely that in certain circumstances the information that is important to your study may involve illegal or stigmatized behaviors, such as illegal drug use, HIV status, a history of violence or abuse, or sexual orientation. Just as in providing counseling or other services to these clients, conducting research with them requires a special level of trust in order to ensure that meaningful and accurate information is exchanged. In these situations it may be beneficial and reassuring to secure a Certificate of Confidentiality (COC) from the National Institute of Health and other Health and Human Services (HHS) agencies at http://grants.nih.gov/grants/policy/coc/, in order to provide participants some protection when participation in your study may surface illegal or stigmatizing information.

Your research does not have to be funded by NIH or HHS in order to qualify for a COC. COCs were created by the National Health Services Act in 2002, to protect information that is gathered as part of a research process from forced disclosure in legal and other proceedings. The certificate of confidentiality ensures that data cannot be subpoenaed or disclosed during legal proceedings and offers an additional layer of reassurance and protection to study participants. For social workers and other "mandated reporters" it is important to note that despite having the COC you are still required to report suspected child abuse or the threat of imminent harm to self or others.

Many of the aspects of confidentiality that we have just discussed have direct implications for a third ethical concern identified by Tutty, Rothery, and Grinnell (1996), which is information management (IM).

Information management

In this era of electronic communication and portable data, information management issues for research studies are more important than ever. The data derived for your PBR purposes should be treated as carefully as client records of any sort – perhaps more carefully. Client records can be secured in locked file drawers or in protected computerized data-systems. And while the latter are vulnerable to hackers, nothing is more easily accessible than a two-inch "flash drive" with all your data, lost or left carelessly about. Consequently, in your PBR studies, efforts should be made to ensure that any identifiable data be handled only by those directly involved in your study, who have completed a human subjects sensitivity training (available online such as www.citiprogram.org), and who have the express approval of the IRB when appropriate. Computers holding data should be password protected, and care should be taken not to leave information open on screen when others are in your office. Any original notes or transcriptions should be filed without identifying information, with identification codes being kept in a separate location from the data.

As a further protection, client research data can be destroyed after an approved period specified by your IRB (usually between 3 and 5 years), but should be kept in this secured manner while they are in existence. Original or "raw" data have to be maintained for a specified period so that if anyone wants to question your findings or your analysis, you have the original data that can be used to show the foundations of your analysis and interpretations.

As information technology continues to evolve we urge you to be mindful of how secure data transfer systems are before you use them. For example, when fax machines first came into use, it seemed like an ideal way to quickly transfer client records or research information. However, it soon became apparent that once material was faxed you often did not have control over who retrieved the information from the fax machine or what happened if a wrong number was accidentally dialed. Similar considerations concerning the security of server platforms and password access should be given to e-mailed data.

RANDOMIZED CONTROLLED TRIALS AND THE ETHICS OF WITHHOLDING TREATMENT

An additional ethical concern rarely raised in academic research considerations is central to PBR studies. More specifically, it is the common research strategy of withholding treatment for purely research purposes. Since PBR studies by their very nature occur within practice settings, and have as a major underlying assumption that when they are in conflict, practice imperatives have a higher priority than research imperatives, it is hard to imagine a PBR study situation in which withholding treatment or services for comparative purposes is ever warranted. In "gold standard" RCT research, this strategy is employed in its most extreme form through the use of control groups which receive no intervention whatsoever.

To be fair, researchers who employ this strategy do not do so out of cruelty or a desire to punish, but because they honestly believe that the intervention might be harmful and the absence of intervention either beneficial or harmless. In pharmaceutical studies where a potent drug may be more harmful than a placebo, this logic makes sense. Our position is that in PBR such a practice is not justified.

While from a research design perspective the internal validity of a study may be considerably stronger with a control group against which to test your intervention, this is rarely ever the case from a practice perspective (see our related discussion in Chapter 4). In PBR studies, however, the same logic may be ethically employed when due to limited staff resources a waiting list situation may occur. In these instances, if they consent to it, those on the waiting list might be included in your study as a comparison group. However, since it is unlikely that the determination of who was being seen and who was on the waiting list was based on random assignment, those on the waiting list would not meet the technical criteria for a "true" control group.

More likely, current clients were selected to receive services either based on the severity of their symptoms or situation, or based simply on when they applied (i.e. first come first served). In either case, the way the clients were assigned to the wait-list condition would not warrant their being used as a control group with the internal validity protections that would accompany random assignment to the two (or more) groups. As a result, definitive cause–effect inferences about the effectiveness of treatment or services could not be made. Approximation to such might be strengthened by studying the demographic characteristics and presenting problems of both groups to see whether they are comparable. However, since the process of randomization maximizes the likelihood of comparability on every possible dimension (whether studied or not), only those studies in which random assignment was the basis for who was in an intervention group and who was not meets this standard, everything else is approximation.

Again, however, since PBR studies are by nature occurring in practice settings then those participants joining your study are likely there because they are trying to access services of some kind. Delaying services in the name of research is an ethical violation from a PBR perspective.

It could be argued that if you are going to have two groups, then why not randomly assign clients to the two groups in order to conduct a more internally valid study? But there are reasons we don't think random assignment is a feasible or ethical option for PBR. First, random assignment does not represent a standard practice protocol. In fact, an essential element of practice expertise is based on an opposing principle – that of matching the type and severity of client need to appropriate services. Second, as practitioners our mandate is to provide as full a range of services as resources allow. As a consequence "rationing" of services for purely research purposes violates practice norms.

A final ethical barrier to the use of control groups is that in "gold standard" RCT studies, the only way to assure that the "integrity" of the research design is maintained involves seeing to it that those in the control group do not receive services elsewhere during the time of the study and similarly that those receiving treatment or services do not receive additional services elsewhere. Hence, both groups must be carefully monitored for research purposes.

Even if you are employing a wait-list approximation to an RCT, it requires preventing those on the waiting list from accessing comparable or other types of treatment while they are waiting. If an opportunity arose to try a potentially helpful adjunct therapy or herbal treatment, then either they would not be permitted to try the treatment or they would be excluded from the study, and thus potentially lose their place on the waiting list. It's easy to see how each of the foregoing scenarios necessitates artificial treatment settings in which both practitioners and service recipients are required to compromise their interests to satisfy research purposes.

Finally, we contend that even though we might learn the most about the efficacy of any intervention through an RCT, the very tight monitoring of all participants creates false and distorted results, since when the treatment is integrated into regular use such tight monitoring would not be maintained. In that sense, one might even question whether the "gold standard" is really a gold standard after all.

Leaving that fundamental epistemological question aside, chances are we can learn as much from repeated comparison studies as we can from a controlled trial. In comparison studies, one group in the study may not be receiving treatment because they are on a waiting list, or they may be receiving the regularly available treatment in that practice setting. We call the regular treatment protocol the "treatment as normal" condition for research purposes. In treatment as normal comparisons we are looking to see if the change in the group that receive the treatment we are studying is greater (or better) than the change in the group that receive our regular treatment. So for PBR we recommend creative approaches to comparison studies so as to uphold our social work value of service and our ethic of beneficence while building knowledge for practice.

INSTITUTIONAL REVIEW BOARDS

As we have discussed throughout this chapter, institutional review boards or their equivalents represent organizational oversight of research studies, monitoring proposals, protocols and procedures to ensure that benefits outweigh potential risks and to ensure that individuals are not harmed or exploited through the research process. The structures, composition, procedures, and meeting frequency of these committees vary considerably. For example, in research centers and teaching hospitals IRBs may meet weekly whereas in family service agencies and child welfare settings, they may meet on an as needed basis depending on the volume of research studies within their organization.

While IRBs have varying structures and compositions, they do often include researchers from a range of disciplines, a community member, and an advocate for vulnerable populations. The IRB checks all aspects of the interaction between you the researcher and your participants including any recruitment materials or procedures that you plan to use, the way in which outreach will be conducted, the informed consent procedure and matters relative to the risks and benefits of the study along with the way in which data will be protected and remain confidential or anonymous as appropriate.

Complaints occasionally heard against IRBs include their being overly bureaucratic and that they overstep their role by acting as a gatekeeper to what can and cannot be studied, especially disallowing more sensitive potentially controversial studies at a higher rate than non-sensitive studies (de Grunchy and Lewin, 2001; Ceci, Peters and Plotkin, 1985). In medical settings, they have been known to favor RCTs and quantitative studies and treat qualitative research as "unscientific". Fortunately, the field of nursing has a strong tradition of qualitative research and it is often nurses who sustain methodological pluralism in these settings. Finally, some have suggested that IRBs are more about protecting the agency or hospital against litigation than protecting clients or patients. Clearly, IRBs represent an evolving organizational effort to solve a set of research-related problems. In fact, the study of IRBs themselves and the decisions that they make has become a burgeoning area of research (Sieber, 2004).

Whatever their merits and liabilities, IRBs are a necessary and important part of the research process. And while, occasionally their requirements feel like an obstacle to conducting your well-intentioned and practice-relevant study, it is always better to be safeguarding the rights and interests of service recipients rather than unwittingly sacrificing these for the sake of knowledge. For this reason we encourage you to become familiar with the IRB procedures and to secure IRB approval before beginning any PBR project.

SOME ADDITIONAL ETHICAL/METHODOLOGICAL CONCERNS

There are three additional ethical concerns that have as much to do with research methodology as with the protection of human subjects. Still, they warrant our attention here. The first concerns the relationship between research subjects and the researcher. Although it's an issue in every type of research involving human subjects, this relationship is especially open to exploitation in qualitative research (Goodman, 2001; Tutty, Rothery, and Grinnell, 1996). In some respects, these issues are familiar to all social work clinicians who are trained to monitor their own counter-transference responses to clients in order to protect clients from placement of workers' needs above their own.

Because PBR involves combining the roles of practitioner and researcher however, doing so confounds the ethical concern to some extent. Here again, the intentional blurring of the lines between research and practice in PBR requires a special awareness on the part of the practitioner-researcher in response to the age-old and ever-useful question *cui bono?* If you never took Latin and are unwilling to Google it, it simply and profoundly means "who benefits?" The IRB will ask that question of your research proposal, but you should ask yourself the question before it even gets there. We'll say more about this in relation to qualitative research studies a little later.

Two additional ethical/methodological concerns relate to every kind of research – whether qualitative, quantitative, RBP, PBR, RCT, NPR (just checking), etc. These concerns are more about maintaining the integrity of the knowledge-building and dissemination process. They go to the fundamental question of what research is all about. And whether you see yourself as a practitioner-researcher, a research-based practitioner, a post-positivist, a critical theorist, a phenomenologist or a herpetologist (again, just checking), the reason one does research is to make discoveries and learn things rather than to reinforce one's own biases. Simply stated, it's about seeking or getting closer to what is in some sense "true".

This emphasis on "truth-value" has implications for prior research studies as well as your own. Thus, in reviewing prior research, every researcher and every practitioner-researcher is ethically bound to be inclusive of all populations (Dodd, 2009) and to give balanced attention to studies that either support or refute one's own biases and expectations. Similarly, in analyzing and reporting your PBR findings, the ethical principle of veracity or truth-telling is equally important.

Earlier, we suggested that the nature of the relationship between researcher and research subject adds a particular layer of ethical concern in qualitative studies where the researcher and the respondent engage in an active, potentially intense and sometimes ongoing dialogue (Goodman, 2001; Tutty, Rothery, and Grinnell, 1996). Thus, as a practitioner-researcher conducting a qualitative or mixed-method study, it can be very difficult for you as a practice-based researcher to separate your clinical goals from your research goals. On this point, Goodman (2001) comments that, "the desire to reach out to help informants seems to be a reasonable response for people trained as helpers" (p.299). If the participants in your study are also your clients then this impulse is magnified, and you have to weigh your clinical responsibility with your research responsibility. It is for this reason that sometimes it is better not to engage your own clients in original qualitative data collection. Instead, you might interview the clients of colleagues, and ask a colleague to interview your clients. If you do wish to study the experience of your clients you may also choose to rely on more unobtrusive methods, such as retrospective qualitative data mining of your case records instead (Epstein, 2010).

More generally, in situations where the research process promotes or solicits intense emotions it is important to remember that the voluntary nature of participation provides for people to stop an interview at any time or even to withdraw from the study if they are not comfortable. Research ethics also require that you have appropriate referrals available (both inside and outside your agency) should the respondent become distressed during or after data collection. While we are emphasizing the possible negative impact of research involvement of service recipients, we would be remiss in failing to acknowledge that agency clients often welcome the opportunity to provide both quantitative feedback about the services they have received and qualitative feedback about their own experiences – even if they are painful ones. Hence the empowering aspects of client involvement in research and "giving voice" to clients through qualitative research should not be overlooked. In their zeal to "protect" human subjects, IRBs sometimes ignore this potentially positive link between practice and research.

A further ethical issue we would like you to be aware of as you review prior literature and/or construct interview or survey questions for your PBR study is to be aware of the full range of your potential respondents so as to try to generate categories that are inclusive, exhaustive and non-offensive to all potential participants. For example, typically, researchers have not asked questions related to sexual orientation, and as such study findings cannot shed light on ways in which lesbian, gay, or bisexual individuals are impacted by an issue (Dodd, 2009; Boehmer, 2002). Hence, Boehmer (2002) conducted a MEDLINE search and found that out of 26,554 articles located in a search of "breast cancer" only 6 considered lesbian, gay, bisexual, or transgender (LGBT) individuals as part of the analysis. A valuable opportunity to learn about the ways in which LGBT individuals are similarly or differently impacted by breast cancer was lost because of the lack of inclusion either in the study questions or analysis.

Moreover, adjusting "traditional' response categories on intake forms and research questionnaires can be an important way to communicate inclusivity to participants, if only binary gender categories are available then instantly any gender nonconforming individuals feel excluded from your study. Similarly, restrictive racial and ethnic categories minimize people's experiences of race and ethnicity and may make some people feel invisible to the researcher. Relationship status categories could be adjusted to be more specific and thus affirming of a full range of relationships asking to specify both relationship status and partner gender (same gender, opposite gender, transgender or gender queer, and other) when appropriate.

If in doubt, pilot-test your questions with different people before you settle on your final wording or response categories. Also, a Community Advisory Board (CAB) or Research Advisory Committee (RAC) composed of a range of potential participants (including LGBTQ and other marginalized individuals) should be formed to advise throughout the process and ensure cultural competence, inclusivity, and sensitivity (Dodd, 2009).

The final ethical issue for you to consider as you conduct your PBR studies is the ethical principle of veracity or truth-telling as it relates to the honest and accurate disclosure of your research results. It is possible that the findings of your study will not reflect positively on your practice or your agency. There is a temptation in these situations not to report the findings at all, or even to "spin" the results into a positive light. Upholding the ethical principle of veracity it is important to report even these potentially negative findings since much can be learned from them. In fact, we suggest because it has been true in our own research experience, that as a practice-based researcher you learn the most from those findings that are counter to your expectations. And we would contend that your clients will benefit most from those findings as well since they often highlight previously unidentified needs, practices that call for improvement and/or objectives that are not achieved. When these unanticipated findings are honestly shared, social workers in similar practice situations may recognize aspects of their own practice in your reported study and use the information as the impetus to monitor or change their own practices and/or programs.

SUMMARY OF KEY CONCEPTS

In this chapter we briefly discussed the distinction between values and ethics. We discussed key events that were the catalyst for attention to research ethics, including the Nuremberg trials, the Tuskegee syphilis study, and the Belmont report. We explored the three primary areas of concern in research ethics, namely informed consent, confidentiality, and information management. We debated the ethics of randomized controlled trials and the emphasis of not withholding treatment in PBR unless it is a necessary part of routine practice procedures, perhaps because of a lack of resources. The purpose and constitution of institutional review boards (IRBs) was also explored. Finally, we drew your attention to three additional ethical/methodological concerns that are particular to qualitative research and to PBR studies conducted by practitioners. The potentially intense nature of the PBR relationship calls for inclusiveness of your protocols and procedures, and the imperative to accurately and honestly report your findings even when they do not always reflect positively on your agency or your practice. Indeed, that's the way we learn the most from PBR.

Part 3

Analyzing and interpreting results in PBR

Chapter 11

Analyzing qualitative data in PBR

Purpose

The following two chapters introduce some of the basic techniques that you can use to analyze your PBR data. In them, we discuss how to approach your analysis with both qualitative and quantitative data. For analyzing quantitative data we provide a discussion of some very basic statistics. But there is no reason to fear. Our purpose is to demonstrate that anyone can do data analysis. In fact, we will try to convince you that as a practitioner-researcher you are uniquely placed to ask the most practice-relevant questions of your data. Likewise, in Chapter 13 which focuses on interpretation of findings, we will argue that you are in the best position to understand their practice implications as well.

In this chapter we review some basic steps involved in analysis of qualitative data, while in the next chapter we explore quantitative data analysis. As in previous chapters, all that is required is that you keep an open mind about your capacity to integrate research ways of thinking with practice ways of thinking (which is actually the ideal way to approach PBR data analysis). Our hope is that you will leave these chapters excited about the prospect of analyzing data related to your practice and equipped with beginning skills to do so.

INTRODUCTION

Throughout this book, we have made reference to the historic notion of social workers thinking of themselves as ill-equipped to conduct research and not especially interested in doing so – in other words, that they are "research reluctants" (Harder, 2010; Epstein, 1987). Perhaps the most significant barrier to more research self-confidence is the spectre of data analysis. After all, social workers collect and interpret information all the time. What they don't routinely do, however, is interpret this information systematically. This applies to individuals but most especially to aggregates of individuals. In other words, they make generalizations all the time but in doing so follow no explicit rules. This chapter and the next are about "rules" for systematic analysis of data. And while the rules are not that difficult to follow, they greatly improve our capacity to make valid generalizations in order to learn from our data.

In the next two chapters we hope to coax you out of any reluctance that you might have, and even tip you in the direction of curiosity and eagerness. It's been known to happen (Hutson and Lichtiger, 2001). And, since the reluctance about which we speak is especially true of quantitative (number-based) analysis, then we will begin by looking at qualitative analysis. Think of it as the establishing trust and confidence part of the relationship.

Given that social workers tend to think of themselves as "relationship" and "process" people rather than "number crunchers" or "bean counters", we will begin our discussion of data analysis with the non-numerical, qualitative sort. This seems logical since much of qualitative data is based in relationship and draws on the logical and information-gathering skills that you routinely use as part of problem assessment in your work with clients. Once we have considered some of the ways in which you can organize and analyze your qualitative data, then in the next chapter we will embark on our consideration of quantitative data, slowly and gently!

Now we know that at this point you may be thinking that this is all fine for some people, but in your agency setting you may have access to a research consultant to do your analysis so it doesn't really matter for you. Or if you do any research after you graduate, you can always hire a research consultant to do the analysis for you. Or your research professor may express interest in working with you in the future and she or he can handle the data analysis part.

Well, using a research consultant/analyst is fine and may even be necessary in some studies (see Chapter 13). However, we still think it's important for you to have a basic understanding of data analysis because even if you intend to use a research/statistical consultant to assist you, having a foundation knowledge of analysis can help you to ask the right questions and create a mutually accountable partnership that together very effectively develops and executes a plan for understanding your data. We have seen far too many practice-based and practitioner-initiated studies in which the data analysis was simply turned over to a consultant and which did not satisfy the knowledge-development interests of the practitioners involved in the study conceptualization and data collection.

So let's begin with what you need to know about ways to "clean", organize and analyze qualitative data. Just as there are many schools of social work that vary to some extent but teach much the same thing, there are also various "schools" of qualitative analysis, including grounded theory, phenomenology, constructivism, heuristic research, feminist criticism, narrative analysis, textual analysis, etc. And while proponents of these different approaches make much of their differences, what is common to all is that they all involve the "content analysis" of non-numerical data. That's what this chapter will emphasize.

Then, in the next chapter we will discuss "cleaning", organizing and analyzing quantitative data with some descriptive (very basic, one variable) statistics, and a few inferential (slightly more complicated, two or more variable) statistics. Take a deep breath. You may even enjoy this!

PREPARATION FOR QUALITATIVE ANALYSIS: BEFORE YOU BEGIN

As we discussed in Chapter 7, qualitative data involves the analysis of information that is not in the form of numbers. It may be in the form of recorded spoken, written or recorded words and/or behaviors either directly observed or captured in pictures, videotapes, etc. In fact, it may include virtually anything that is non-numeric. The way in which you receive or retrieve your data may vary via interviews, observations, open-ended questions in self-administered surveys, etc. But once you have collected the data, the first step in the analysis is always to organize what you have into a manageable format. You want to know when, where and from whom the data was gathered, as well as what it says and, ultimately, what it means.

As we discussed in the previous chapter on ethics, however, you don't want the data to be attributable to identifiable individuals if someone comes across the raw data by mistake, or later in a finished report or publication. For that reason you should always develop a coding system as quickly as possible so as to separate the identifying information from the qualitative data itself, i.e. the actual record of the data (the videotape, interview notes, written responses, etc.). You should then store the data in one location and the code key in another to preserve confidentiality as securely as possible.

The organizational system that you use to keep track of your qualitative data should allow you to easily trace and locate a particular part of your data when needed. A numeric or alpha-numeric system that helps you to create chronological patterns can be helpful. For example, you may number your participants 1, 2, 3, etc., and then use alphabetical letters if you have more than one interview, observation or session recording. So you could note each separate observation or interview of those participants as A, B, C, etc. In this way you could locate notes related to your second interview with your third subject, as the notes would be marked 3B.

Once you have created coded identities for the participants and the particular interaction that your notes are related to, then you can create a detail track of the notes from the exchange. For example, within the written transcript of the data you can number each line or each paragraph depending on the size of the data and level of detail in the document. Using this system, the quote in Box 11.1, which came from the 35th – 39th line of an interview with your first subject in their first interview would be noted as (1, A, 35–39).

There are computer programs including Microsoft Word that will write the number of the line for you as you go along so that you can just make the notes and not worry about adding in the numbers. As with the literature review, create your own system

BOX 11.1   QUALITATIVE TRANSCRIPT EXAMPLE: A CLIENT
DESCRIBING HIS DEPRESSION

Subject 1   Meeting A

35   *I just felt really lost like this black cloud would come over me and I couldn't*
36   *do anything.* [slight chuckle] *I couldn't move off the couch. I couldn't move*
37   *and yet my head would race. I couldn't see anything clearly and I couldn't get*
38   *it to slow down. I was stuck on the couch unable to move with my head just*
39   *spinning.* [deep sigh]   (1, A, 35–39)

to identify themes in the data (e.g., metaphors for depression, severity of depression, denial of depression, etc.), and then start using it right away so that you don't become overwhelmed trying to organize a large amount of data once it has all been gathered. As you find new categories, e.g., precipitants of depression, efforts to decrease depression, etc., you can add them to your coding scheme. Jot these themes down because they will come in handy when you begin actually coding the data.

Verbal and videotapes need to be transcribed before you can begin to analyze them. Transcription is a repetitive process that involves recording in written (usually typed and stored on a computer) form what you believe you hear from a tape recording or see in a video recording and then re-playing the tape/video to check that your written record is accurate. Sometimes you may have to listen to or watch a section many times before you are confident that you are accurately rendering the exact exchange. The written transcript looks like the text in Box 11.1. Although this process can be time-consuming it is absolutely essential since your study findings will be derived from the transcription record of your interviews or focus groups.

You will need to determine whether you would like to transcribe the data yourself, or whether you will hire someone to do the transcription for you. Whoever is doing the transcription should be sure to include details in the audiotape that provide information, such as pauses, silences, inaudible words, coughs, laughs (awkward and authentic), and changes in voice tone or volume. You should note the degree of and any changes in background noise or particular noises like the sound of a chair scraping. In the example in Box 11.1, you can see how the participant's slight chuckle and deep sigh were noted in brackets. This is important because each of these may provide clues later in the analysis phase of the process.

Although transcription can be tedious, paying someone to do it can be quite costly and if the transcriber is not conscientious, valuable data can be lost. In addition, transcribing the data yourself provides a leg up on the actual data analysis. So unless you are transcribing purely mechanically and mindlessly, you will begin to identify themes, categories and sub-categories in the raw data as it is transcribed. Using qualitative software (to be discussed later in this chapter) allows you to attach codes to these categories and themes as you transcribe the literal content.

One final part of pre-analysis preparation is to ensure that your data are as complete as possible. Whether you are gathering written data from meeting minutes or case records or are analyzing transcriptions of video- or audiotapes, make sure that the written representation that you use as the basis of your analysis is as complete as it can be. That means making sure that when you are transcribing, all non-verbal cues, such as coughs, laughs, or long pauses are included in the transcribed document. These may prove to be highly significant in the analysis.

Likewise, from qualitative case records look for as much detail as possible including the equivalent of non-verbal communication, for example worker representations of the client's emotional state. If your data are not complete then you do not know whether you have systematically left out something important. If you do, it can negatively impact the integrity of your findings, their interpretation and their usefulness to practice.

THE PROCESS OF ANALYSIS

Once you have all of your data transcribed you are ready to begin the analysis phase of the process. Box 11.2 outlines six essential steps for you to navigate in the process of analysis. While the steps are presented in a linear format, in reality the phases may overlap in some places and you may loop back to earlier steps if necessary as you go along.

Step 1: Establish your purpose

As you can see from Box 11.2 the first step is to establish the purpose of your analysis. This stems directly from your problem formulation and your underlying reasons for conducting your study in the first place. Given that in qualitative analysis there is often a large volume of information to sort through, it is important that you have a very clear idea of the questions that you want your analysis to focus on, so that you can listen, watch or read with a clear sense of purpose. Although, this is not to say that you shouldn't be open to discovering the unexpected from your data, just that you should know what the specific questions are that you are hoping to answer.

Step 2: Developing an overall sense of the data

The second step in the qualitative analysis process is to listen, watch or read through your data uninterrupted from start to finish. In this phase you are not focused on the specific details of the data but rather on getting an overall general sense or feeling about the data set as a whole. For example, you want to identify what is the overall tone of the data. What emotions and behaviors are expressed in the data? Are there any emotional or behavioral connections or patterns that pop out at you straight away? These are the same kinds of questions that you ask yourself when you do an assessment. And just as when doing a clinical assessment, it is important to record these first impressions in a journal to be reviewed later in the analysis. You can then see whether your initial impressions were upheld once you delved into the details of the data. You can also ask yourself if they varied and why you think that might be.

What's different about qualitative data analysis, is that the data are right in front of you and you can work at your own speed, systematically and carefully without the client or client group saying something else. In other words, you can control the flow of data as you reflect upon its meaning. That's the good part. The not-so-good part is that, unlike an assessment interview, you can't ask clients what they meant by their prior statement or if they can say more about the reasons for saying it.

Step 3: First level coding

In Step 3 you do first level coding, which is sometimes referred to as first order coding. First level coding is when you manually or using a software program such as Atlas.ti, NVivo or NUD*IST begin to code your data by identifying meaning units, which are chunks of text that represent different categories of information relevant to your study. You are asking on a concrete, raw level, what does the text say? At this phase you are not offering any interpretation of what you think the text says or what the text means; you are categorizing what it actually says into chunks of ideas represented by categories. You are also recording how frequently the meaning chunks that are identified appear. Are there some meaning chunks or phrases that appear several times, or do they appear in isolation?

We feel strongly that since the data are gathered about your practice, you are in the best position to identify and understand the meaning chunks that emerge. However, it does require maintaining a fine balance between imposing what you expect to see/read and utilizing your understanding of the practice context to interpret the information provided. There is a degree of intimacy with the data collected that is only available to you as the practitioner who collected it.

If you have a theoretical foundation informing your work then the way that you create these meaning units should be consistent with your theory. That doesn't mean that you look at the data with the intention of supporting your theory but that you use it to test whether your theory is consistent with the data. In other words, you note those text chunks that fit into categories that are identified by your theory, but you also identify text content that is not yet identified by your theory. In this way you are testing the categories created by your theory to see whether or not they are present in your data and whether there are sets of ideas or "chunks" of data that are not captured by your theory. So for example, while your theory about a client's depression may focus on "loss" associated with your client's situation, you would as well want to record data about "gains" associated with the situation. Similarly, many studies of adults caring for their elderly parents emphasize "caregiver burden" but it is equally important to note what psychological benefits caregivers receive for their efforts.

If you do not have a theoretical foundation guiding your study, but are instead working purely inductively, your challenge is to develop a theory from the data itself. This approach is known as "grounded theory" and involves identifying and naming categories that seem to emerge from the data and form the foundation of your theory development. Of course, it's never possible to be completely atheoretical in looking at data, but in grounded theory that is the ideal.

In all forms of PBR data analysis, however, you always come back to the central question of how do the data inform practice? What can we learn for practice? In this way you continue to keep your practice-based research question central in your mind as you conduct the analysis. Here again, saying "isn't it interesting that the client says this or that" is not enough. What is important is how does it inform your understanding of the client's situation, and/or what you are going to do about it.

If you are collecting data about more than one client, during this phase of qualitative data analysis you are looking not only within an individual person's response but also across different people's responses or reactions to see where they are similar and where they are different. You can even tabulate or create some basic quantitative tallies of the number of times particular themes emerge. It is important to note not only the frequency with which an idea arises but also the strength or force with which the idea is raised. At this stage, you also look for patterns to establish the extent to which particular types of words or phrases are used. For example, are the comments or actions vague or specific, strong or weak, formal or informal, consistent or inconsistent, happy or angry? You should also listen or read for whether there is a change in energy or sentiment or emotion at any point. If there is a change in energy, tone or sentiment you may want to try to identify what the "trigger" was in the client's situation or in what you did or said that may have been responsible for that change.

Step 4: Second level coding

Once you have established what the data says through first level coding, then you try to interpret what you think the data mean. If you are using a theory then during second level coding you are testing the extent to which your data do or do not support your theory. You are also looking for other interpretations of meaning that extend beyond your theory or particular nuances related to when, for whom and how the data support your theory.

It has been argued that intimate knowledge of the subject or the practice setting can interfere with an "objective" interpretation of the data (Padgett, 1998). However, again, we believe that your intimate contextual knowledge of the data can actually serve as a strength rather than a weakness, and increases the level of sophistication and nuance as you search for meaning within the data. That is why we strongly urge you to analyze your own data even if it is in partnership with someone else. Working closely with someone else can be a protection against bias but, even if you are working alone, you should be open to alternative theories and interpretations of data. PBR is not about selectively looking for evidence to support your practice theories. It is as much about discovering you are wrong as discovering you are right.

If you are working from a grounded theory approach then it is during this phase that you begin to consider whether there is a theory about clients' needs or problems that is beginning to emerge or aspects of a theory that are emerging that are relevant for practice (Glaser and Strauss, 1967). You begin to name the relationships and patterns that the data seem to convey. You also pay attention to the extent to which the findings seem to reinforce "practice wisdom" or run counter to it.

This is especially important if your data involve cultural differences that have not heretofore been studied. So for example, generalizations about African-Americans may not apply to clients from the West Indies. Likewise, generalizations about American-born Latinos may not apply to recent immigrants from Mexico. Gender-based theories may not apply to GLBT clients and generalizations about GLBT clients may not stand up to scrutiny when you look at differences within this category.

At this point it may be good to go back to your first impression notes from Step 1, the initial listen, watch, or read to see whether your understanding of meaning is consistent with or different from those initial impressions.

Step 5: Seeing the forest not the trees

During qualitative data analysis it is important to allow time for your ideas about the meaning of the data to gestate and evolve. Just as we can gain important clinical insight when we allow ourselves to consider a case on a subconscious level, so we can gain important analytical insight the same way. You may have noticed that often if you re-read data with "fresh eyes" and through "different lenses" you notice things you didn't notice before. Or, you may interpret something differently from the first time you looked at it. Maybe you see a new angle. (A typo in our first draft suggested that you may see a new "angel", which may also be true!)

Stage 5 is about building time into your analysis schedule to consciously allow that renewal process to unfold, so that you don't get hung up on a few particular details (trees) within the data but rather have a sense of the whole picture (the forest). Sometimes it even helps to envision yourself standing back from your data and seeing what you imagine as emerging or even jumping out at you. Very often your first "off the cuff" or "gut" responses to the data reflect the emergent and overarching themes that are embedded in the data. Trust those responses, but once you have articulated them see how consistent they are with multiple chunks of data. Those chunks that aren't consistent may lead you to modify the themes slightly.

Step 6: Reporting results

We will discuss interpretation of results and dissemination of findings more fully in Chapter 13, but it is important to note reporting results here as an important step in the data analysis process since we see it as integral to the PBR mission. In PBR we do not do research for its own sake but rather to inform one's own practice and the practice of others. Given this, then your analysis is never complete until your results have been shared with relevant parties so that they may inform practice. Whether you disseminate findings internally or externally, to other clinicians, agency administrators, consumers, or the broader social work community, it is important to share your findings so that others can learn from your experience, and collectively we can inform practice. Who knows, others may even be inspired to conduct their own PBR study so that they can test their own findings against yours.

BOX 11.2 STEPS FOR QUALITATIVE ANALYSIS

STEP 1
Establish the purpose of your analysis (or interview)
Purpose: To establish the purpose of the research or the analysis.
Task: To ask questions of the data just as you would in an assessment (or with statistics).

Box 11.2 continued

STEP 2
Read/watch the data straight through
Purpose: To get an overall sense of the data set.

Task: Time may not permit but when possible before you begin your analysis read, watch or listen to the data in full, straight through with an open mind and without judging it to get a sense of the overall data set – all cases or interviews at once.

STEP 3
First level coding
Purpose: Look for patterns and prevalence.
Try to read energy or emotion.
Look for shifts in energy, sentiment or intensity.

Task: Identify categories (meaning units) and begin coding.
At a <u>concrete</u> level what does the text SAY?
Note similarities and differences.
Note patterns that arise (frequencies, orders, magnitudes).

STEP 4
Second level coding
Purpose: To interpret the data.

Tasks: Interpret the data on a more <u>abstract</u> level – begin to identify what you think the text MEANS.
Begin to determine whether the findings support your theory or whether there is a theory that you think is beginning to emerge.

STEP 5
See the forest not the trees!
Purpose: To identify the "big ideas" in the data.

Tasks: Try to stand back and listen to the patterns or the "big idea" in the data.
What is the main message that the smaller messages are conveying?

STEP 6
Reporting results
Purpose: To communicate the results to key stakeholders.

Tasks: Focus on a few key findings (too many points reduces their impact) Focus on the strongest patterns or the most salient question that you started with. Summarize the main ideas and use quotes to illustrate and highlight your points. Too many quotes can be distracting. Find the ones that most directly exemplify the themes you wish to identify. You can also create frequency tables for identified themes. You can create charts to illustrate patterns. Finally, you can incorporate frequencies into your discussion of findings by indicating that "5 out of 7 clients reported that they required assistance with … " and then illustrate with a few direct quotes.

QUANTIFYING QUALITATIVE DATA

As you plan your data analysis you may decide that although your data are presented primarily in qualitative form, there are some quantitative questions that you would like to ask of it. Alternatively, it may become apparent as you move through Steps 1 to 5 in the analysis process that some themes or ideas are emerging more frequently than others and you would like to convey the magnitude of those differences to your audience. Where the qualitative database involves 10 or more, you might report the percentages that responded in a particular manner. In those instances it can be beneficial to "quantify" your qualitative data by tallying the frequency with which themes or ideas emerge in order to create a frequency table, or to create percentages for reporting purposes (i.e. what percentage of the respondents reported that the professor they had was instrumental in their favorably changing their opinion towards research, and what percentage reported that the textbook that they used was the pivotal factor in engaging their love of PBR). You may also create a matrix that shows the frequency of different ideas separated out by the different categories within a variable. Table 11.1 provides an example utilizing a matrix that indicates the agency auspice of the practitioner and the quantity of specific ethical issues identified.

TABLE 11.1   Example of a qualitative data matrix

| Agency auspice | Ethical issue identified | | |
	Autonomy % (N)	Confidentiality % (N)	Patient best interest % (N)
Public	40 (12)	26.6 (8)	50 (15)
Private not-for-profit	30 (9)	56.6 (17)	73.3 (22)
Private for profit	26.6 (8)	33.3 (10)	70 (21)

BOX 11.3   SOME HELPFUL HINTS FOR QUALITATIVE ANALYSIS

- Gather complete data
- Be organized!
- Create a coding system right away
- Keep notes on your reactions and impressions as you review the data
- Build time into your analysis for your ideas about the data to percolate
- Beware of bias!

BEWARE BIAS IN YOUR ANALYSIS

A final note of caution as you conduct your qualitative analysis is to beware of your own sources of bias. Often, as you develop your PBR questions you may be tempted to assume that you "know" what you are going to find. But in actuality, one of the foundations of PBR is the assumption that you do not know what you are going to find. To successfully conduct PBR studies you have to be open to being surprised. For this reason you should remind yourself as you undertake your analysis that it is important to know what questions you are going to ask of your data (hence our emphasis on establishing your purpose), but definitely not what you are going to find. You should know what variables you are interested in, and even what relationships between variables you are interested in, but it is not possible to know what those relationships will be until you have studied them.

SUMMARY OF KEY CONCEPTS

As the first of two chapters on data analysis, this chapter focused on the process of qualitative data analysis with an exploration of each phase of a 6-step data analysis process that spans from establishing the purpose of the analysis to reporting the results (see Box 11.2). Key preparatory steps prior to beginning qualitative analysis are also discussed including transcription and the importance of creating complete data. Finally, the idea of quantifying qualitative data through the creation of frequency tables and charts is described. Throughout the chapter we tried to convey both how manageable we believe qualitative data analysis is for social work practitioners, and also the important and unique position you as a practitioner-researcher are in with regards to analyzing and understanding data related to your practice. The next chapter will explore quantitative data analysis for PBR studies with the same emphasis.

Chapter 12

Analyzing quantitative data in PBR

Purpose

OK, this chapter is the one you've been dreading. It's all about quantitative data analysis, the aspect of research that social workers seem to fear most. In the chapter, we review levels of measurement (you survived the original discussion in Chapter 8), we gently introduce very basic descriptive statistics, we adventurously explore a few more advanced inferential statistics, and we conclude with a reader-friendly discussion of how to conduct relatively simple quantitative analyses with a commonly available statistical software package called Statistical Package for the Social Sciences (*aka* "SPSS"). Keep breathing, it's one of the few requirements.

As with the previous chapter on qualitative data analysis, we will try to dissuade you from a lifetime membership in the "reluctants club" and persuade you that quantitative analysis is understandable, manageable, important to know how to do as well as how to critically comprehend, and can even be fun! It's a tall order we know, but our many years of successful and enjoyable teaching of research to social workers, convince us that it can be done.

INTRODUCTION

Building upon your knowledge of qualitative data analysis developed in the previous chapter we will apply similar ideas like generating complete data, establishing purpose, and looking for relationships – only this time, doing it with numerical data. First, we discuss "cleaning" your data, which is related to the idea of complete data that we explored in our discussion on generating a usable qualitative database. Second, we need to review the levels of measurement already discussed in Chapter 8. Then, we introduce descriptive statistics, which are quite literally the numbers that describe your data – one "variable" or dimension at a time. We call the analysis of these individual variables "uni-variate analysis". Such analyses might be used to describe the demographic characteristics of your client population or the frequency with which they require different kinds of services, or the percentage that achieve positive outcomes of one kind or another.

After discussing uni-variate statistics, we ease cautiously into slightly more complex statistics that allow you to look at relationships between any two pairs of variables – such as gender and service requests, race and services received, diagnosis and mental health outcomes, etc. We call these "bi-variate" relationships. Bi-variate analyses are even more exciting than the uni-variate kind because they help you consider associations between different aspects of your clients or your practice via what are called "inferential statistics". These statistics allow you to infer whether any of the relationships you find can be assumed to reflect true relationships in the population you are studying, and how strong they are.

We discuss these bi-variate analyses and statistics using a common computer software package easily available to social work practitioner-researchers called "SPSS". SPSS is routinely available in every university. If you're reading this book in conjunction with a research course you are taking, we're sure your instructor has access to it and can provide you with it as well. Otherwise, you may have to purchase the program directly from SPSS (the student version is much cheaper but each database is limited to 50 variables, which sounds like a lot but can mount up quickly).

Whatever statistical package you use, the logic behind the statistics is the same and will be explained so that you can use any quantitative data-analytic program that either you are comfortable with or that is easily available to you. Just in case you need some reassurance, in addition to teaching research to MSW and doctoral social work students, we also have many years of experience conducting statistics and SPSS workshops and consulting with practitioner-researchers on this topic. And, we promise that there is nothing in this chapter that we have not successfully explained to social work practitioners who have in turn successfully used the concepts, skills, techniques and research technology in conducting research on their own practice.

PREPARATION FOR ANALYSIS: ORGANIZING YOUR QUANTITATIVE DATA

In the previous chapter we introduced the idea of organizing your qualitative data so that you could easily identify and track who or what it was about and when and where it was gathered, as well as of course what it said about them. A very similar process is required with quantitative analysis. It is important that you organize your data systematically so that you can develop a coding system that keeps the "raw data" (i.e. the original format in which the data came) separate from the identity of those individuals, groups, organizations or other units of analysis from which the data were gathered.

Just as with qualitative data the first step is to develop a distinct identity code for each person, case, or other unit in your data. For anonymous data (where there is no identifying information anywhere on the data) then the ID number still serves importantly as a way for you to link your raw data and the information that you enter into a computer based data program like Excel or SPSS. This is important because you can then easily check that the data have been entered correctly, something we will discuss in greater detail in a moment.

For confidential data, where it is possible to trace your raw data back to particular individuals, families, groups or organizations, then the ID code serves as a valuable layer of identity protection, whereby you create a code sheet with each data source assigned an ID number and their identifying information. That information and code number must be kept in a locked location separate from the actual data set. In this way, if someone accidentally comes across the code sheet they would not be easily able to link the data source to the data or vice versa. Once you have given all of your raw data an ID code then you are ready to set up your database in a computer program, which will greatly facilitate the conduct of your analysis. Of course, you could do it by hand or with a hand-calculator but that would be so much more cumbersome and time-consuming – even with a relatively small data set. Even then, you would not be able to do anything more statistically sophisticated than uni-variate frequencies, percentages or averages. But if you are interested in looking at relationships between variables and determining their statistical significance (and trust us, you will want to) the computer is the way to go.

SETTING UP A DATABASE

Many of you are already familiar with the Excel computer program, which offers a simple way of entering quantitative data into the computer and developing some statistical analysis. Excel can be a really useful program, especially if using it gives you more confidence in your ability to conduct quantitative analysis. If so, then start with Excel or any other basic quantitative data analysis program that you are familiar with.

In our discussion, we are going to explain how to set up a database using SPSS, arguably the most widely used quantitative data analysis program available precisely because it is both user-friendly and can do everything from the most simple to very complex data analyses. In addition, the manuals that come with SPSS are excellent guides both to how to use the program and to how to understand the "output" it produces. For starters, if you are familiar with how an Excel spreadsheet looks then SPSS will not seem too unfamiliar. Like Excel, SPSS has cells in which you can enter data, but unlike Excel it also has a "brain" for each cell, which keeps track of the value code for each category and "knows" what each number in the cell represents. So, for example, if you have a variable related to whether or not a client is living independently, you may create a value code of 1 for living independently and 2 for not living independently. Then, when you compute your analysis using SPSS those values are represented in the charts and tables produced. This can be useful for a number of reasons, but it also means that different people entering data can easily check what the numeric value is for a particular item and you can be sure that you are all using the same code. If you want to, the value codes that you create can be printed out in a codebook or quickly referenced by clicking on "variable info".

Box 12.1 provides step-by-step instructions for setting up a database (sometimes called a "data file" or "data shell") using SPSS software. However, since SPSS is already in its 19th edition and is constantly being updated, the directions in Box 12.1 may change slightly as SPSS evolves. But don't worry, each version of SPSS has a comprehensive tutorial section available that walks you through many of the key features of the program if you need an introduction or a reminder. And it rarely changes much from version to version. Moreover and most important, the basic logic of it all remains the same.

So, regardless of SPSS updates and new statistical "bells and whistles", our example in Box 12.1 should provide the basic framework to help you to set up your database. As you will see, there are a series of simple but systematic steps to be followed and decisions to be made in order to prepare the database for your data. Box 12.1 walks you through the different steps including assigning a short label (8 characters maximum), a longer explanatory variable name, codes to represent different responses, and a number to represent missing values. We will briefly describe each of these steps here, but it will be most useful for you if you can open the actual SPSS program and walk through the steps in Box 12.1 with the program open in front of you.

Once you have opened your database you need to tell the "brain" of the cell what the numbers you put in that cell represent. You do this by filling out information for each cell. The information needed for each cell is laid out clearly in the variable view. The same 10 questions need answering for each variable that you want included in your database. The questions appear clearly across the top and you have an opportunity to add as many variables as you choose down the left hand side. Once you add a variable name default values drop into many of the answer spots. In some cases you will want to keep the default value, while in others you will want to change them. Once you understand what each piece of information represents, then you will be able to decide. It can be a bit tedious, especially if you have many variables, but it is certainly not difficult.

Since each cell represents a different variable or dimension in your study, you are assigning the categories or "qualities" of the variable. First, you have to give the variable/cell a nickname a short 8-character name that can fit easily along the top of the data view replacing the word "var", which appears as the default. Make the name something that you can recognize as representing that variable, and that you can locate in a long list. Try not to use question numbers, such as q1, q2, etc. as your variable name, because when you are conducting analysis this variable name will not prompt you about the meaning of the variable and you'll have to keep referring back to the data-gathering instrument to remind yourself what the question was. You can imagine if you have an intake instrument with 75 questions on it, just naming the cell "q43", will not help you to know what variable that cell represents.

The second column of variable information represents "type", and asks you to select from a "drop down" menu of different variable types, such as numeric, date, dollar, string. (A string variable is one that uses words not numbers. It allows you to enter written words but limits the type of analysis you can run with these data.) The default for this choice is numeric, which will almost always be what you want. But note that if you select numeric you will not be able to enter any non-numeric characters into the cell. For example, you won't be able to enter B3, or C4, since these entries would be alpha-numeric. You also can't put in $23, since that has a non-numeric dollar sign.

The third column requires information about the "field width", or how many digits or characters you wish to enter into the space provided. The default width is 8, which is more than enough for most numeric variables that you will be entering. On the rare occasion that you wish to enter numbers that are greater than 8 digits, you can click on the arrows to add digits. However, if you are entering string data (i.e. words rather than numbers) into the cell you may want to make a substantial increase to the field width, since 8 characters is very limiting when you are entering words.

The fourth column is "decimal" and is asking how many decimal places you would like visible in your data view. This is one place where we recommend changing from the default, which in this case is for 2 decimal places to be visible to 0 decimal places. Our reasoning is that the majority of the variable information that you enter will be whole numbers 0, 1, 2, 3, etc. not fractions 2.25, 3.46, etc. If you put in a whole number with the decimals set at 2 then the number that appears in the data window is 0.00, 1.00, 2.00, 3.00, etc. As you can imagine that having a wide array of unnecessary zeros visible on the data view can be confusing, so switch the setting to zero unless you are entering data in fractions. If you wish to change a large number of decimal values at once you can use the "copy and paste" function, so that you don't have to manually change the setting for each individual variable.

The fifth column is entitled "label" and is an opportunity for you to write in the long-hand version of what the variable information represents. In a sense it is the key to the nickname assigned in the first column. Be as specific as you can in the label, so that if you take a vacation, with your permission, one of your colleagues could open up your data set and easily know what each variable represents. For example, if you named your variable age, then your variable label should specify "age in years" or "age in years and months". It will also help you when you return to remember what it was you were thinking in creating this data set.

The sixth column is where you assign values to your variables. If you recall from Chapter 8 when we discussed levels of measurement, the values for nominal variables are arbitrary and for ordinal variables are merely ranked, whereas those for interval and ratio represent an actual number or score. The sixth "value" column is where you assign those arbitrary values, both so that you are consistent as you enter your data and so that someone else can pick up for you midway through if necessary. This is where you might assign English speaking client = 1, Spanish speaking client = 2, Russian speaking client = 3, other = 4. In this way if you entered a 2 into the variable cell then it would represent a Spanish speaking client, a 1 would represent an English speaking client, etc. Similarly, for an ordinal level variable you may decide that 1 represents strongly agree, 2 represents agree and so on or that 5 represents strongly agree and that 1 represents strongly disagree. The values are still, in some sense "arbitrary" but you have to enter the data consistently with each "strongly agree" response being represented by the same number.

If you have an ordinal scale that utilizes the same answer categories for several questions, or a series of yes/no answers, then there is good news. You can enter the values that you wish to use in the column for one variable and then click on the cell and "copy" it, just as you would in a Word document. You then highlight all of the cells that you want to have the same values and you click "paste". The values should be filled in for each variable that you selected, although it is always a good idea to open a few just to check that it worked as you expected.

The seventh column is titled "missing". This is where you assign a numeric value that you will enter if a participant has left the information question blank. This happens when occasionally someone skips a question either purposefully or by accident. This can also happen if a participant fills out the front side of a questionnaire without realizing that they are also supposed to complete the backside of the page. While it is true that you could just leave the cell blank, assigning a missing number helps you first to check that you have a complete data set, since each cell is filled. Second, you can assign a reason for the missing value noting a different missing value for not available, not known, and not answered. And, third, assigning missing values means that blank responses can be pulled out of your analysis, so that the frequencies and percentages that are generated represent a proportion only of those responses given. Again, there is good news! If you wish to assign the same missing variable number(s) to several variables, then you can copy the missing value cell that you wish to use and paste it into the other cells that you want to have the same missing value. Be careful to make sure that the number you use for missing data is not a possible answer option for the variable. For example, if there are 12 different answer choices for presentation problem labeled from 1–12, you should not make 9 your missing value, since it is a possible response.

The eighth column is titled "column" and refers to the column width of the variable that will be visible in your data view. There is rarely a reason to adjust the default column width, which is set at 8. However, in the rare case when you need to, you can make the columns narrower or wider to fit your needs selecting a smaller number for narrower and a larger number for wider.

The ninth column "align" refers to how you would like the information to align in the cell in the data view – the three options provided are align right, align left, and centered. The default is align right, but you can experiment with each and then select the one which is most comfortable for you.

The tenth column is called "measure" and refers to the variable's level of measurement. The column has a drop down menu with three answer options:

- scale
- ordinal
- nominal.

Scale refers to both interval and ratio level variables, and ordinal and nominal should hopefully be obvious to you by now.

All of the above sounds complicated and arduous, but when you actually start doing it and get the hang of it's really kind of fun. In fact, completing all ten columns for each variable that is included in your data set, you will be surprised at how quickly you become familiar with the columns, and since often you are either utilizing the default value or copying and pasting values, you can quickly become proficient at creating the shell of the data set.

Once you have set up the parameters for each variable then you are ready to take a test run to check that you really have entered all of the variables that you need to, in the order that you need to, with all the information that is needed. To do this select any survey, or case record, or data sheet from the total set for which you have created your data shell to enter and see if it works. Remember to start with the assigned ID number and move through the rest of the information. Make sure that you have not accidentally skipped a variable or a potential response.

One common mistake to be aware of is for lists that ask a person to "check all that apply". For example, how did you hear about our program: (1) flyer, (2) friend, (3) email, (4) referral? Check all that apply. Each option has to be set up as its own separate variable in SPSS with a yes/no designation (i.e. was it checked yes or was it checked no?) These types of questions cannot be entered as one variable in one cell of the data set, because if someone checked two or more boxes you would have to choose which value to enter into the cell. Therefore, you have to set up a separate cell for each answer option with the response choices of yes/no to show whether or not that particular answer option was checked. Once you have checked your data shell works for your test case record or survey, and you have made any necessary adjustments then it is time to enter your data.

BOX 12.1 CREATING A DATABASE USING SPSS

1 Open SPSS
When you open SPSS the first screen looks exactly like a spreadsheet with numbers down the left hand side and variable labels along the top. The variable labels are denoted by "var" until you assign them the label that you want them to represent.

2 Find the tabs
At the bottom of the screen, you will see two tabs one that is called "data view" and one called "variable view". If you toggle between the tabs you will see that the data view is the spreadsheet that you opened on, and the variable view is a blank space available to assign characteristics to your variables. N.B. variables are listed along the top in the data view and down the side in the variable view.

3 Set up a data file to match your needs

For each cell/variable you have to define

- Name – 8 characters or less
  - This name will appear in the data view in place of the term "var"
  - Name the variable something that identifies it to you or others. However, you are limited to 8 characters. Something with less than 8 letters is easy e.g. ethnicity, but more complicated need a shorthand e.g. swyears may represent years of social work practice, or livind may represent whether they are living independently or not
- Type – (number, date, string, etc.)
  - This indicates the type of information that you will enter into the cell. Most of the time you will be entering numeric data and so will select numbers, but occasionally you may want to enter a date. String variables refer to written non-numeric information. You may have a string variable if you have an open-ended question on your survey and you want to type the responses into he database. Entering a variable as a date or string limits the type of analysis that you can run.

Box 12.1 continued

- Width – (default is 8)
  - Refers to the number of digits or characters that may be entered into the cell. It is rare that you wish to enter numbers greater than 8 digits into the data set. However, you may wish to adjust it for string data.
- Decimals – (default is 2 decimal places – adjust to 0 if appropriate)
  - Decimals refers to how many decimal places are in view on the spreadsheet (in the data view). While the default is to show 2 decimal places, it is often good to adjust this to 0 when appropriate, as otherwise it is quite distracting to have a lot of .00s showing in your view.
- Label – allows you to more fully explain the variable name
  - Since the name had to be shortened to 8 characters, label provides you with a chance to explain what you meant in the name! Be sure to give full information in the label so that others can understand the name that you assigned. E.g. the label for "swyrs" might be Years worked in Social Work (not just years worked in SW, as someone may not be familiar with SW).
- Values – assign numeric values to responses
  - This is where you are able to explain what the numbers in your database mean. You assign values to each potential category for each variable. E.g. you may assign democrat = 1 and republican = 2.
  - Click on the value box, Click on the small gray box, type in the value and value label that you want to assign, Click "add", when complete Click continue
  - Copying values – when several variables have the same values assigned e.g. no = 0, yes = 1. You can copy the value label from one variable and paste it to the other variables.
- Missing – assign value for answers with no response
  - Often there are questions that are left blank. It is important to note that the data is missing from the raw data so we assign a missing value, which allows those responses to be left out of the analysis. You can assign any number as the missing value as long as it is not a possible response to the question for which you are assigning it. It can be good practice to use 9, 99, 999 or 9999 depending on possible answer responses.
- Columns – the width of the column on view in the data view
  - This refers to how wide the column width is as you are looking at the spreadsheet. Unless you have a particular need it is easiest to leave this set at its default of 8.
- Align – how the data are aligned in the cell
  - Data in the cell can be aligned right, left, or center. The default is right for numeric and left for string, but you can adjust as you prefer.
- Measure – the level of measurement of the variable
  - The three options provided are nominal, ordinal, and scale. The default is scale, but you can adjust as appropriate.

Box 12.1 continued

4 Enter data
- Once you have defined each variable in your data set then you are ready to enter data
- Use arrows to move around the cells
- Enter each case all the way through (so entering data across a row)
- Save at the end of each case
- If there is an error, click on that cell and type the correction – it automatically overwrites the existing entry

---

ENTERING YOUR DATA

Just as precise transcription is a crucial foundation for qualitative analysis, so precisely entered data is crucial for quantitative analysis. However, take our word for it – it is virtually impossible to enter data perfectly with no errors even for people who do this all the time. (This is why we will be discussing cleaning the data to correct for any mistakes very shortly.) Entering data into SPSS is just the same as entering data into Excel: you put your cursor in the cell and then type in the data for that cell. If you make an error put your cursor on the cell and type the correct data, there is no need to delete the original entry, as there is an automatic overwrite.

While there is a temptation to get faster and faster as you enter data and become familiar with the codes and the rhythm of the information, try not to go too fast. It is very easy to make mistakes by entering in the wrong box or hitting the wrong key on your keyboard. Remember you are doing this to learn more about your clients and your practice from the data, so you need to make sure it accurately represents them. Also, make sure that you "save" at the end of each survey or case record. Losing a day's worth of data entry is very distressing (unfortunately, we also know this from first-hand experience!). Finally, back up all of your data in more than one place and keep it in a locked location so as to preserve confidentiality.

CLEANING THE DATA

Once you have entered all your data, then it is time to do what we call cleaning the data, which involves checking that you have not made any mistakes in data entry. While both you and your computer are very smart and ideally good friends, even good friends occasionally have communication breakdowns. Thus your computer cannot know whether you have assigned an incorrect value – it takes a real live person to do that! Unlike good friends, computers are there to do exactly what you tell them to and if you enter data incorrectly, the computer won't know it.

Do not assume that your data are correct, if anything assume that there are occasional and sometimes big mistakes since, no matter how careful you are, it is highly unlikely that there are no mistakes at all in your data set.

Box 12.2 walks you through the steps of data cleaning. The goal is to act as a detective to find any errors that might exist, so first you look for obvious errors and then you double check some cases to make sure that there aren't hidden errors. You may also find errors when you do your first data runs on the frequencies associated with each variable. Thus if a yes/no variable, which is generally coded 1 Yes and 0 No shows some respondents with a value coded "2", then you know something is wrong in your data entry. Once the data are clean then the fun really begins because you can start to explore your data to see what they say.

ANALYZING THE DATA

Just as with qualitative data, when you analyze quantitative data you are looking for patterns and relationships that can inform you about your clients or your practice. It is also important to keep your research questions uppermost in your mind. You don't want to get caught running tests for tests' sake. Being clear on the purpose of your study and having a plan for analysis will help you to choose the most efficient and effective way to answer your questions with the data you have.

In quantitative analysis there are two different types of statistics that you can use to explore your data, descriptive statistics and inferential statistics. Descriptive statistics describe a single variable. They help to summarize the numbers and depict

---

BOX 12.2   CLEANING YOUR DATA

- "Eyeball" the data fields for any answers that look out of place e.g. a 33 among a sea of 3s.
- Run frequencies for all variables.
- For each variable check for any answers where the value is not one that you have defined. For example, if political affiliation has two choices (values 1 for democrat and value 2 for republican) but 5 cases are assigned a value of 3, then there is an error. Check the data set to find these 5 cases. Then match their ID number and recheck their original survey or raw data.
- Repeat that process for any errors noted.
- Once all of the frequencies fall in line then pick ten cases arbitrarily to check the values. (If possible have a second person do this so that fresh eyes see the entries.) If all 10 are spot on, great. Pick 5 more just to make sure. However, if you find several errors, change them and then double-check 10 more. When you are reasonably sure that the entries are correct it is time to start the analysis.

---

patterns created by the numbers, literally describing the data. Once you understand what each individual variable revealed then you might begin to look at relationships between variables using inferential statistics, which analyze relationships between two or more variables.

Descriptive statistics

To describe your data you can use frequencies and frequency tables that show how often your clients responded to a particular question (variable). Frequencies count how often each response occurred for a variable. Box 12.3 walks you through the steps to generate a frequency table for each of your variables using SPSS. If you wanted to do more outreach and were looking at how your clients came to hear about your program, then your results might show that 26 (out of 40) of your clients said that they heard about your program from a friend, nine were referred by their health care provider, and only five said that they heard about it from a flyer. This would represent a simple report of the frequencies of the one variable.

If you have more than 10 cases then it is customary to report percentages rather than frequencies so that you can easily see the proportion of your respondents that answered a question in a particular way. When you do report percentages it is also customary to report the actual number of responses that the percentage was created from, referred to as the N. The same results reported as percentages would be that 65% (N = 26) of your clients heard about your program from a friend, 22.5% (N = 9) were referred by a health care provider, and only 12.5% (N = 5) saw a flyer.

Another thing to keep in mind is when reporting results from an SPSS printout it is important to report the "valid percent", since this represents the proportion of responses without including missing responses (i.e. those respondents or cases in which you have no data for that particular variable). In essence, the valid percent represents the percentage response of those that answered the question, or for whom a response is available.

As you may have seen yourself in research articles that you have read in the past, it is often useful to illustrate your results in table form, especially if you want to report the frequencies for a large number of variables. We will discuss this further and provide examples in the next chapter on dissemination of results. "Research reluctants" often avoid tables while research "dorks" like ourselves often immediately go to the tables because we know that's where we can get a big bang for our buck. Over time, the more experience you have in doing this sort of thing the more comfortable you will become.

MEASURES OF CENTRAL TENDENCY

Once you have described the frequencies of your variables, the next step is to look at how the scores clustered. Measures of central tendency refer to the statistics that we use to see where the "middle" of the data falls. You may not realize it, but you are familiar with the idea of central tendencies because you frequently use it when you refer to "averages" or make generalizations about what is "typical". In quantitative

BOX 12.3   GENERATING FREQUENCIES IN SPSS

- Click analyze.
- Click descriptive statistics.
- Click frequencies.
- Send the variables that you would like to analyze to the right hand box.
- Click on statistics and select the measures of central tendency and measures of dispersion that you would like to analyze.
- Click on charts and select whether you would like bar charts or a histogram with a normal curve. Then click continue.
- Always report <u>valid</u> percent as this excludes missing cases, or the cumulative percent.
- When reporting the mean always report the standard deviation as this provides the reader with information about how spread out from the mean the scores were.

analysis we use these terms more precisely in the form of specific statistical measurements and additional facts surrounding them. All of this makes for greater precision in understanding and communicating your findings. The three measures of central tendency that we routinely use are the mean, median, and mode.

Before we continue, it is a good idea for you to refresh your memory about levels of measurement. As you may recall from Chapter 8, levels of measurement (nominal, ordinal, interval, and ratio) refer to the way in which response categories are created for a variable. If the responses simply represent categories without a specified order then they are nominal, if they have an order but arbitrary numerical representation, then they are ordinal, if they have equal distance between numeric categories then they are interval, and if they have all of those features and a true zero then they are ratio. Keeping in mind the level of measurement is crucial as we move forward because it determines which statistics are appropriate for use. Some statistics are appropriate for some levels of measurement and not others.

The mode

The mode represents the most frequent or most popular or most typical response. It answers the question "which answer was given most frequently?" and can be reported for nominal, ordinal, interval, and ratio data. In the event that there is a tie and one or more responses are the most frequent, then we refer to the variable as being bi-modal (two modes) or multi-modal (three or more modes).

The median

The median response is the answer that falls in the middle of all the answers where 50% fall above and 50% fall below when the responses are laid out in order. If you ask seven clients how many children they have and their responses were 1, 2, 0, 4, 2, 2, and 1, then to calculate the median you would line them up in order: 0, 1, 1, 2, 2, 2, 4 to find that 2 is the middle response or median. If you have an even number of responses then you take the middle two responses add them together and then divide by two to get the median. So, if you had an eighth client with one child, then you would have: 0, 1, 1, 1, 2, 2, 2, 4 – the middle two numbers are 1 and 2. You add them together to get 3 and then divide by 2 so that your median number of children is 1.5. More often than not, the median is an approximation because there is no exact 50/50 split. But the median is as close as the distribution can get to that.

The median can be reported for ordinal, interval, and ratio data, but is not useful for nominal data since there is no rank-order that can be used to lay them out in order. So for example, you can meaningfully say what the "modal" diagnosis in your school-based client sample is ADHD, but it would make no sense at all to say that ADHD was the median diagnosis.

The mean

The mean, commonly known as the arithmetic average, is perhaps the most familiar of the measures of central tendency. The mean is calculated by adding all of the scores together for a particular variable and then dividing by the number of scores available. Using the example of number of children from above for 7 respondents the numbers were: 0, 1, 1, 2, 2, 2, and 4. If we add those scores together we get 12 and then divide by the number of scores (7), we get a mean of 1.7. If we add the extra score (1 child) we get a total of 13 to be divided by 8 scores, which gives a mean of 1.6. The mean can only be used with interval or ratio level data, since the numbers have to have an actual meaning in order for them to be added together in a meaningful way.

One thing to be aware of with the mean is that one extremely high or extremely low score can pull the mean in a particular direction, so if the eighth person had 10 children rather than one it would have inflated the total to 22 (0, 1, 1, 2, 2, 2, 4, 10 = 22) and made the mean 2.75. Therefore it is a good idea to report the median and the mean. Think about it, if Bill Gates decided to get an MSW and we surveyed the annual income in your class, his income would vastly inflate the impression that an "average" income would suggest. For this reason when there are "outliers" on a variable like income, or length of stay, or numbers of treatment sessions (i.e. a few or a single case with really extreme scores quite different from the rest) we generally use the median to express the central tendency. The reason is that the median is not affected by extreme scores. Thus if the wealthiest person in your class earned $30,000 a year or $30,000,000 a year, the median income would be exactly the same.

It is also good "research practice" to always present the standard deviation along with the mean. The standard deviation tells you how spread out the scores are. If the scores are all clustered very tightly together then the mean is a good representation of the responses (shown by a low standard deviation). But, if the scores are all spread apart (a high standard deviation) then the mean is probably not a helpful representation of the scores. The mean can be represented by the symbol x and the standard deviation by SD. A report of results describing the mean would read "the mean number of children was $x = 2.75$ (SD = 1.25). More precisely, because of how the standard deviation is computed, this finding would tell you that 66.6% of your client families have between 1.5 (mean minus s.d.) and 4 (mean plus s.d.) children. This is why the SD is often represented in the form of +/–.

The standard deviation is known as a measure of dispersion. Measures of dispersion test the question how dispersed or spread out are the scores? Another commonly reported measure of dispersion that is useful for you to report is the range. The range tells us the highest score, the lowest score and how far apart they are. So we would report that our clients had a mean of 2.75 children (SD = +/–1.25), with a range from 0–4.

You can see that you can provide a good deal of information about your clients and your practice simply by analyzing the individual variables in your data set to look at the frequencies, percentages, mode, median, mean, standard deviation and range. However, we still might want to know if there is a relationship between two or more of our variables and for that we need inferential statistics; for example is there a relationship between family size among the homeless and success in locating adequate housing? The answer may seem obvious but there could be circumstances that make it easier for people with larger families to secure housing than those with fewer children or none at all. That's why we do research. The answers are often not what we expect.

INFERENTIAL STATISTICS

While there are a vast number of inferential statistics that you can apply to your data, most of those available fall beyond the scope of this book. We are going to focus on the three most commonly (and easily) used statistics to give you an idea of what is possible. We will introduce the chi-square, the t-test, and Pearson's correlation. In time you may want to read statistics books such as Weinbach and Grinnell (2010) *Statistics for Social Workers* (8th edition) or Craft (1990) *Statistics and Data Analysis for Social Workers* (2nd edition), or take classes to learn about even more ways to analyze your data. This has been known to happen when practitioner-researchers get fully engaged in the process.

In this book, however, we will focus on bi-variate analyses, which look at the relationship between two variables. As you become more advanced you may learn multi-variate analyses, which look at the relationships between three or more variables. These more sophisticated analyses are especially good for "explaining" relationships between two variables or "controlling" for the effect of a third variable but we'll leave that to future and/or other available research texts.

For now, let's stick with bi-variate relationships. As we saw with measures of central tendency, not all statistics are appropriate for all levels of measurement. In fact, there are specific rules about which tests work with which types of variables. Therefore, when conducting bi-variate analysis the first thing that you have to do is to determine the levels of measurement of the two variables that you want to analyze. In the case of nominal variables you also want to know if they are dichotomous (have only two categories) or not (have more than two categories). Remember however, that you may have only men or only women in your sample but the variable gender (like any other nominal variable) must have at least two categories. Otherwise, it couldn't vary either in principle or in fact.

Once you know the level of measurement then you can decide the appropriate statistic using the chart in Box 12.4. To determine the statistic, find the level of measurement for your first variable down the side and then read across the top until you find the level of measurement for your second variable. For example, if you are looking at the relationship between age (measured in years – interval) and whether or not an advanced directive has been completed (measured as Yes or No – nominal). You would look down the side for nominal to represent advanced directives and then along the top for interval to represent age. You would see that it is a 2-category nominal and so would find the appropriate test in the bottom left hand box as the t-test. Similarly if you wanted to test the relationship between gender and having an advanced directive (two nominal level, dichotomous variables), then you would read along and find the appropriate test is the chi-square. We will discuss the specific tests in more detail now.

Chi-square

The chi-square (χ^2) statistic is used to analyze the association between two nominal level variables. It works by comparing the expected distribution (how you would expect scores to spread out if there was no association at all between the variables) and the actual distribution. There should be a minimum of 5 subjects in each cell, for the test to work correctly. In some cases you can "collapse" or combine categories to achieve compliance with this. However, that would necessitate a simple "recode" function that SPSS provides.

Perhaps you are studying intake data for 40 of your client population and you are wondering whether there is a relationship between prior substance abuse history (yes/no) and prior incarceration (yes/no). If there were no association between prior substance abuse history and prior incarceration, then by chance alone you would expect the clients to spread equally among the boxes of a two by two table (called a cross tabulation or cross tab), as shown in Figure 12.1.

BOX 12.4 SELECTING THE APPROPRIATE STATISTICAL TEST

Level of measurement	Nominal (2 categories)	Nominal (3+ categories)	Ordinal	Interval
Nominal (2 categories)	Chi-square			
Nominal (3+ categories)	Chi-square	Chi-square		
Ordinal	Chi-square Mann–Whitney U	Chi-square	Spearman's Rank	
Interval	T-test	ANOVA	Spearman's Rank	Pearson's Correlation

		Prior substance abuse	
		Yes	No
Prior incarceration	Yes	10	10
	No	10	10

FIGURE 12.1   Cross tabulation (example 1)

But if there was an association between prior substance abuse history and prior incarceration then the clients may distribute as shown in Figure 12.2.

		Prior substance abuse	
		Yes	No
Prior incarceration	Yes	25	3
	No	2	10

FIGURE 12.2   Cross tabulation (example 2)

The chi-square statistic tests the difference between the expected distribution and the actual, empirical distribution to see how far apart they fall. It also provides a numerical score known as the chi-square statistic, which tells us the likelihood of there being an association between the two variables. It also tells us whether or not the chi-square is statistically significant, which refers to whether or not the results happened by chance. The significance level represents how certain you are that the difference that you found between groups is real and exists. (Or how certain you are that the lack of difference you found is accurate.) The significance level is known as the p-value and has been described as the "mathematical probability that a relationship between variables found within a sample may have been produced by a sampling error" (Weinbach and Grinnell, 2001, p.88). That is, you reached your conclusions but it was because your sample didn't really represent the population you were hoping to represent. Sampling error means that there is always a chance that our conclusions are wrong, so the probability or significance level tells us what the chance is that we are wrong!

The significance level is usually framed as how certain you are that you can reject the null hypothesis, which is the hypothesis that assumes there will be no difference between groups. With our chi-square this would be the assumption that there was no association between the variables to generate the expected distribution.

In social work research, we tend to use a significance level of .05 as our standard to determine whether or not there is statistical significance. If you set your significance level at .05, then any number smaller than .05 is considered to be significant e.g. .02 or .006, whereas any number greater than .05 is considered to be not significant e.g. .08 or .12. So, what does the .05 level really tell us? It tells us that it is likely that any difference we found does actually exist. In fact, we are 95 percent sure that the outcome did not happen by chance, but rather that the difference is real. Setting the significance level depends on the level of certainty required, if you are just beginning to do research in an area you may want to cast a broader net and use a significance level of .10 (90 percent certainty), so that you catch any possible associations. However, if you need to be more precise for some reason (often the case when pharmaceutical companies are testing a new drug) then you might set the significance level at .01, so that you were 99 percent sure the results didn't happen by chance.

One thing to keep in mind is that because of the way χ^2 is computed, the larger the sample size, the easier it is to get a statistically significant outcome. Hence in our example, if we had a client population of 400 rather than 40, it would take a smaller departure from the expected frequencies to tell us that the finding was statistically significant. Another way to look at it is that χ^2 tells us how safe it is to generalize our finding to a larger, comparable population. The larger the sample size, the more assurance that our finding (whatever it is) is safe to generalize. That's why in epidemiological studies of thousands of patients it may take only a 1 or 2 percent difference in the negative impact of a cancer drug to warrant taking it off the market. But let's get back to social work.

Box 12.5 walks you through conducting a chi-square test using SPSS. It also shows you how to interpret the results and how to report the findings if they are statistically significant. If the result is not statistically significant then you would simply report that there is no statistically significant association between the two variables.

T-test

If you look at the grid in Box 12.4, you will see that a t-test is used when you want to test the relationship between a nominal variable with two categories (dichotomous) and an interval level variable. The independent t-test is used to compare the mean between the two groups. The t-test literally calculates the mean for one group and then compares it to the mean of the other group to see the extent that they differ. Perhaps you want to look at the age of your clients who have advanced directives in place and the age of your clients that don't yet have advanced directives. The t-test calculates the mean age for the group with advanced directives and the mean age for the group without advanced directives and then calculates whether the difference is statistically significant. Box 12.6 walks you through the process of computing and reporting a t-test. As with the chi-square, if you are reporting that there is not a significant difference then you would simply state that there was no generalizable relationship between age and completion of advanced directives.

Box 12.7 gives an example of how to calculate a paired sample t-test using SPSS. A paired t-test works on exactly the same principle as the t-test in that it takes two mean scores and compares them. However, a paired t-test compares two mean scores that are related to each other even for the same person. If you regularly generate a depression score at intake and then again after 3 months of treatment for all of your clients then you could use a paired t-test to generate a mean for all of the intake scores and then a mean for all the 3-month scores and compare the two. You report the results

BOX 12.5 COMPUTING AND REPORTING CHI-SQUARE USING SPSS

To compute:
- Click on analyze
- Click on descriptive statistics
- Click on crosstabs
- Select one nominal level variable and transfer it to the row box
- Select the other nominal level variable and transfer it to the column box
- Click on statistics and check chi-square
- Click on cells and select expected (observed should be checked by default)
- Click OK

To report:
- First look at the top row of the chi-square test box
- Read and report the chi-square value, df, and significance level
- If the results are significant then you must look at the grid and compare actual versus expected counts to determine what may have caused the significance

Example report
The results indicate a chi-square value of 2.02 (df = 1) with a significance level of .0001, which is significant at the .05 level. The scores suggest that the number of clients with a history of incarceration and a history of prior substance abuse is much higher than expected, while the number of clients with a history of incarceration and no history of substance abuse is much lower than expected.

exactly as you would for the independent t-test noting whether there is a significant difference between the two scores and reporting both the mean and standard deviation for each group.

If you want to analyze the relationship between a nominal variable with more than two categories and an interval level variable, then a t-test will not work as it can only process two mean scores. If you review Box 12.4, you will see that if you want to compare the mean scores of more than two groups then you would use the analysis of variance or ANOVA. ANOVA uses the same logic as the t-test but compares and contrasts each different combination of mean scores to see if there is a significant difference between any of them. The Mann–Whitney U test also mentioned in Box 12.4 operates similarly to a t-test but can be used with a nominal dichotomous variable and an ordinal level variable rather than an interval level one.

BOX 12.6 COMPUTING AND REPORTING A T-TEST USING SPSS

To compute:
- Click on analyze
- Click on compare means
- Click on independent samples t-test
- Select your interval level variable(s) and transfer them to the right hand box (testing variable)
- Select your nominal variable and transfer it to the group box
- Click on define groups and enter the values that are represented by the variable
- Click OK

To report:
- Check the Levene's test
- If it is significant read the "equal variance not assumed" line
- If it is not significant read the "equal variance assumed" line
- You must report the t-value, the degrees of freedom and the significance level
- If it is significant you should give the contrasting means for each group along with their standard deviation

Example report
The results indicate a t-value of –2.99 (df = 38) with a significance level of .005, which is significant at the .05 level. The mean age of those clients who had completed an advanced directive (x = 65.48, SD = 13.8) was significantly higher than the age of those who had not completed an advanced directive (x = 54.06, SD = 8.8).

Pearson's correlation

When you are interested in the relationship between two interval level variables then the test that you use is called a Pearson's correlation (it's actually Pearson's product moment correlation or PPMC, but that is too much of a mouthful, so most people call it a Pearson's correlation or even just a correlation). The correlation plots each person's scores for the two variables on a grid (see Figures 12.3a, b, and c) to see if there is a relationship between them. Imagine you are looking to see whether there is a relationship between the age of your clients and the number of physical ailments they noted during the intake. You would anticipate that the older the client is then the

BOX 12.7   COMPUTING AND REPORTING A PAIRED SAMPLE T-TEST USING SPSS

To compute:

- Click on analyze
- Click on compare means
- Click on paired samples t-test
- Select (highlight) your two interval level variable(s) and transfer them to the right hand box (paired variables)
- Click OK

To report:

- The paired t-test is reported in exactly the same way as the independent t-test.

more physical ailments they would report, which would represent a positive or direct correlation (Figure 12.3a). Note that in this context "positive" is not necessarily a good thing. It merely means the higher the score on one variable (i.e. age) the higher the score on the other (i.e. number of symptoms). In other words, the scores cluster in a pattern that indicates that as one score goes up, so does the other score.

Now imagine you are looking to see whether there is a relationship between your clients' hours of sleep reported and their stress level. In this case we would expect a negative or inverse relationship, whereby as one score goes up (hours of sleep) the other score goes down (stress level) (see Figure 12.3b). Here again, "negative" doesn't mean it's a bad thing, merely that as one goes up, the other goes down.

You can tell whether the relationship between variables is positive or negative by looking at the r-value. For a negative relationship the r-value will be a negative number (e.g. $r = -.38$). However, for a positive relationship the r-value will be positive (e.g. $r = .38$). Of course, sometimes the variables we look at have no relationship at all and the scores scatter in no particular pattern (see Figure 12.3c). As with the chi-square and the t-test, the correlation tests to see whether or not the pattern created represents a significant relationship. If it is significant, it indicates whether the relationship is positive or negative and the r-value tells us the strength of the correlation.

The correlation strength can range from .00 to 1.00. The closer the r-value is to 1 the stronger is the correlation and the stronger is the relationship. So in studies looking at relationships among psychological variables (e.g. self-esteem and depression) a correlation of -0.25 is considered not very strong compared to a correlation of -0.85 which would be considered quite strong. We'd expect it to be negative however because self-esteem would be theorized to be inversely related to depression.

In studies looking at more social factors (e.g. years of education and years of incarceration) it is unusual to get a very strong correlation because, unlike the linkages between client self-esteem and depression which are very closely connected, there are many additional factors (such as race) that might affect the relationship between years of education and incarceration. Here again, we would expect a negative correlation

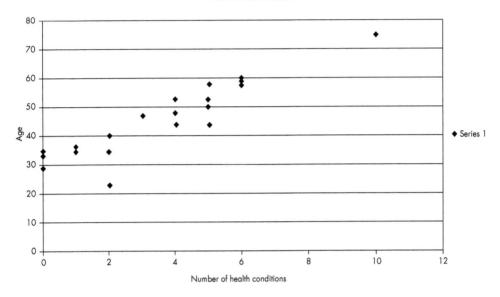

FIGURE 12.3a   A positive correlation

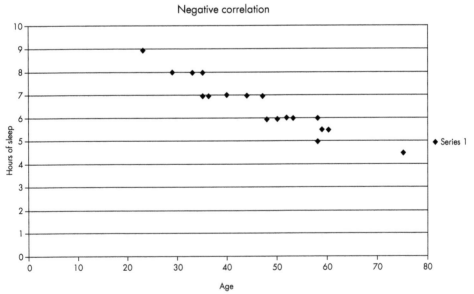

FIGURE 12.3b   A negative correlation

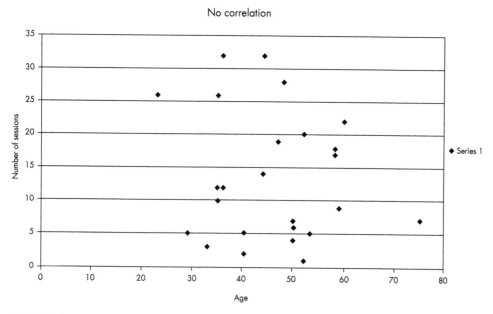

FIGURE 12.3c   No correlation

(the higher the level of education the lower the number of years in prison) but we would never expect an r of 0.80 or above because there are so many other factors that might impinge on this relationship. In this context an r of 0.40 might be considered quite high. In both studies, however, one might wish to conduct multi-variate analyses either to "explain" why self-esteem and depression are inversely related or the conditions under which they aren't. For example, mentally ill adolescents enrolled in a program to improve their self-esteem may improve on their self-esteem scores but remain depressed producing a lower negative correlation than those who did not participate in the program. Wouldn't that be a useful thing to discover if you were running such a program?

Again, you will see from Box 12.4 that if you have one interval level variable and one ordinal level variable, or even two ordinal level variables, then the Pearson's correlation is no longer appropriate. The appropriate test, which works on the same principles as Pearson's correlation is known as Spearman's rank and can be used to test the association of ordinal level variables (see Box 12.8).

SUMMARY OF KEY CONCEPTS

In this chapter we introduced different aspects of quantitative data analysis. We provided a description of how to set up a database using SPSS. We also discussed entering and cleaning data. We emphasized the importance of accurate and complete data, as the foundation for data analysis. Understanding levels of measurement is key

BOX 12.8   COMPUTING AND REPORTING PEARSON'S
CORRELATION USING SPSS

To compute:
- Click on analyze
- Click on correlate
- Click on bivariate
- Select (highlight) your interval level variable(s) and then transfer them to the right hand box (variables)
- Check that Pearson's is checked
- Click OK

To report:
- First look at the Pearson's correlation coefficient (r) and the significance level
- If it is significant you must report the direction (positive or negative) and strength of the relationship.

Example report
The results indicate that there is a significant weak negative correlation $(r = -.16, p = .0001)$ between how often a participant felt unsafe and how much they wanted to discuss safety with their counselor.

to selecting the appropriate statistic, so we reviewed levels of measurement and specified which tests worked with which types of variables. We introduced some descriptive statistics including three measures of central tendency – the mean, median, and mode – as well as some measures of dispersion, the standard deviation and the range.

We also introduced some beginning inferential statistics the chi-square, the t-test and Pearson's correlation, as well as the notion of statistical significance. For each test we described how to run the test utilizing SPSS, and how to report the findings from the test. The notion of statistical significance was introduced and explored in relation to the three inferential tests that we discussed.

We are optimistic that you can follow the step-by-step guides provided in this chapter to run your own analyses, or at the very least to be an informed partner to your statistics consultant. In the following chapter we will discuss how to interpret your findings and disseminate your results so that your study can achieve its goal to inform practice.

Chapter 13

Interpreting and disseminating results from PBR

Purpose

This chapter discusses the final stages of the PBR process. Never has the expression "last but not least" been truer, because without interpretation and dissemination PBR has not achieved its primary objective of informing practice. Naturally, that includes those like yourself who have conducted these studies and other practitioners and potentially academics, researchers, and program funders. So in this chapter we will discuss the importance of interpreting your findings and their practice implications. Here, as in previous chapters, we remind you that the term "practice" is used quite broadly to include multiple levels from work with a single client to program and policy. We will also discuss different ways in which you can disseminate the results to maximize their usefulness (Patton, 2008). After all, PBR is essentially applied research, and it ain't applied research if it ain't applied (you can quote Dodd and Epstein on that).

INTRODUCTION

As we discussed in the two previous chapters, during the data analysis process, whether qualitative or quantitative, you generate the "results" of your study. Some of these may be pleasing and others troubling. Some may leave you underwhelmed. Some may be total surprises. Whatever your findings, they represent empirically-based answers to the questions that you have asked of your data. And for us, that's always better than "going with your gut".

Your central task during the interpretation phase, however, is to "unpack" what those answers mean in relation to your clients and your practice. Once you have done that your goal for dissemination is to share those findings with others who may find them useful for program, policy, or individual, group and/or community practice reasons. So, if your analysis revealed a significant negative relationship between experiences of bullying and school performance, you would consider how this information could influence the development and implementation of supportive and preventive programming. You may then want to share those findings with teachers, parents, program staff and other concerned groups. Likewise, if you found that clients dealing with chronic pain reported less depression when also attending a peer support group, then you may want to recommend peer support groups for all clients with chronic pain and depression. Or, if you found that clients attending your parenting workshop did not seem to be improving their parenting skills, you may wish to review the curriculum and delivery methods. Or, if you found that there was a significant gender difference in program compliance, you might examine how your engagement methods may be received differently by men and by women, and consider possible changes. You may also want to discuss these findings with other clinicians within your agency in an attempt to raise awareness of the need for examination of gender-specific engagement methods.

Ultimately, the goal in PBR is always to apply your findings back to practice. Therefore, interpretation and dissemination of results are conducted from that perspective (rather than the "isn't it interesting" or "what are the implications for science" perspectives). In this chapter we will examine the most effective ways to ensure that your PBR studies serve as a catalyst for practice and program reflection and change. In rare circumstances, PBR findings suggest keeping things just the way they are but that possibility exists as well. Just as research shouldn't be an end in itself, neither should change. (For a research text, this is getting rather philosophical isn't it?)

INTERPRETING YOUR FINDINGS – OR WHAT DO YOUR DATA MEAN?

Unlike a "philosophy reluctant", a "research reluctant" might be tempted to skip over the interpretation phase by asking a research or statistics consultant to "take care of it please". After all, quantitative findings are just a "bunch of numbers" and qualitative findings are just a "bunch of words".

We caution against this relegation of research responsibility for a couple of reasons. First, because as we said with data analysis, no one understands your clients and your practice like you do. This means that you are in a better position than anyone else to interpret or "make sense of" the results. And second, in many ways interpretation of data is an "art" as much as a "science". There is no need to be afraid. In fact, you should be really good at it since in your practice you make interpretive judgments all the time based on things you observe and/or think you observe. Here however, we would submit that subjecting practice to PBR makes your observations and interpretations more systematic and self-reflective. In our opinion, that can only be good.

Given that social work research occurs not in labs but in real-world settings, your task is to interpret the meaning of your findings through the contextual lens of the practice setting and contextual realities from which the data were derived. Social workers are especially good at understanding information within a context, comfortably employing a person-in-environment perspective to practice (Hutchison, 2008; Germain, 1991). In some ways interpretation of data utilizes a similar perspective – perhaps a "findings-in-environment" perspective. Your PBR findings are always derived from a practice context, so having a contextual perspective can help you to better understand what you have found and/or rather what the data might mean.

The critical skill in interpretation of data, therefore, is to reach beyond what is on paper to imagine the findings in context so that you can begin to understand what they are telling you about your clients, your practice, or your program. Who better to do that than you? If you don't believe us then maybe an example will convince you.

In one study that we collaborated on, examining the role and services of a caregiver resource center, the findings indicated that discussing advanced directives with terminally ill patients rarely occurred during the social worker and caregiver interactions (Dobrof et al., 2006). On face value as research consultants it looked to us as though clients were possibly avoiding difficult and painful discussions of advance directives, perhaps because such a discussion would require that they give explicit consideration to dire outcomes.

However, during this study we employed a collaborative data analysis process, whereby the social workers directly responsible for the practice, the director of the unit, and us the "researchers" sat together first to discuss what relationships should be explored during data analysis. Then we would consider both what we thought the results meant, and what we thought were relevant findings to share with others (through academic outlets, articles, presentations, and internal staff meetings). Everyone saw the same data "output" and a summary of the significant relationships along with the direction of those relationships. During one of the collaborative interpretation sessions (we held two or three), the direct practice social workers said – strongly – "we know exactly why advanced directives are discussed only very rarely; it's because that is not one of the topics that we routinely raise with clients". Faced with this "finding", we realized that it wasn't the clients who were avoiding discussing a difficult topic that requires acknowledgement of the difficult potential outcome. Instead, it was the social workers who were doing the avoiding – or at the very least colluding with the client's avoidance.

Another example within the same study involved a clear shift in client demographics, with more clients identified as Latino or Hispanic utilizing the center in the last few months of the study. The director and practitioners quickly realized that this shift was consistent with when a bi-lingual social worker joined the team. Elsewhere, as the research consultant in a clinical data-mining study with liver transplant social workers, Epstein completely missed the practice and policy implications of a "no findings" exploration of liver transplant outcomes for patients with and without histories of substance use (Zilberfein et al., 2001, p.98). That experience taught him to never interpret research findings without inclusion of the practitioners who initiated the study.

Writing about interpretation of findings from the vantage point of a research consultant to a clinical data-mining (CDM) project, but equally applicable to any PBR effort, he comments:

This is when a trusting dialogue between researcher and practitioner is most important and most fully realized. It's also when I learn the most about the contextual influences that practitioners face and the complexity of their thinking about what it is they do. Here both the dialogue between researcher and practitioner and between their empirical findings and their subjective experience are enormously productive and often revelatory. It represents a unique experience for both sets of actors that I find humbling and practitioners seem to find empowering.

(Epstein, 2010, pp.97–8)

REVISITING THE LITERATURE REVIEW

A key task in interpreting the data is coming up with alternative explanations as to what the results mean from a practice or program perspective. And though it may seem like "backtracking", another key task during the interpretation of data phase is to look at what has already been written about your topic and determining the extent that your findings are consistent with or opposed to them. To do this you can revisit your review of literature and look at what the findings were for studies that were similar to yours. You should also look at what you expected the outcomes of your study to be, based on what was discussed in the literature or your theoretical perspective.

If for example, your results suggest that youth development professionals play an important and effective role in disseminating sex education information within your community-based organization and that is consistent with previous studies such as the one by Fisher *et al.* (2010), then you are adding support to existing practice knowledge by confirming that the same holds true in your setting. If in your setting, however, the findings were inconsistent or even inconclusive, you would still be building practice knowledge because we would know that there may be differences dependent on practice setting or client population that need further examination. In other words, program context makes a difference. Then the question would be "why" or "what is it about your program context that makes it different?"

So part of the task during interpretation of the data is trying to offer possible explanations and understandings of your results in comparison to those of others who have studied the same or a similar problem focus. More generally, it is important to think about possible explanations when the results were not as you would have predicted, and/or when the results are "not significant" statistically speaking. As Yegidis and Weinbach (2008) suggest, both significant and not significant findings "can be equally valuable" (p.270). In basic research as well as in applied research, a finding that is not statistically significant is still a "finding" though in the former it tends to receive less attention than in the latter. In PBR, however, it is particularly important to keep in mind that statistical significance is not the same as "social significance". In other words, a statistically insignificant finding may be very significant for practice!

THE IMPORTANCE OF PRACTICE WISDOM
AND PRACTICE INTUITION

While the literature is important as a guide for interpretation, what distinguishes PBR from other research methodologies/perspectives is that PBR "honors" practice wisdom, and practice intuitions are held as equally important in data interpretation as the prior literature.

In our research collaborations with practitioners over the years, particularly during the data interpretation phase, practitioners have a sense of what the data mean that goes beyond the text, as was the case in our earlier examples. There is an instinctive, sixth sense almost, about what the data mean. As a practitioner-researcher, you have a knowledge of your data that a research consultant or statistician cannot have, it is this knowledge which allows you to "see" things in the data that others may miss, or to understand things that others may find confusing. Imre (1985) referred to this as "tacit knowledge" and our prior consultation experience has taught us to take this very seriously. Therefore, we encourage you to be an active participant and an equal partner in the data interpretation process, and to engage your practitioner self fully in the process. It is not just a bunch of words or numbers, it is a different window into your practice world.

DON'T STRETCH TOO FAR – RECOGNIZING
LIMITATIONS

Now that we have encouraged you to get involved, we need to offer a cautionary comment. During the interpretation phase of your PBR study you should not stretch too far. You should be realistic about the limitations of your data and the methods by which they were gathered, and you should state these limitations clearly (and without apology). Here, working in full collaboration with a researcher is often extremely helpful since researchers are by training, if not by nature, cautious. (This paragraph is "evidence" of that.)

Remember, as we discussed in the sampling chapter, you cannot take results from a convenience sample of parents who have children diagnosed with ADHD and assume that your results can be generalized to all parents who have children with ADHD. Similarly, if your sample is drawn from one small community mental health center, then you cannot simply assume that your findings will apply equally to clients of other community mental health settings. There are other things that may limit the generalizability of your findings as well. For example, there may be only a small sample size, or all interviews may have happened in the morning (limiting responses to those who are available during that time and who may have a different experience from those who come to your agency in the afternoon, or evening), you may not have had Spanish translations available, you may have used self-report on surveys that have the potential to elicit socially desirable responses (those that the participants who may feel indebted to you think you want to hear).

All studies, even the most rigorously designed RCTs, have limitations. You have a responsibility to think through as many of those that apply to your study as possible, and to state them clearly, so that anyone interpreting your results can make a decision as to the extent that they have confidence in your findings. On the other hand, you can go too far in stating limitations to the point where you undermine confidence in what you have found. Describing limitations is not an apology, it is an opportunity to demonstrate your understanding of research principles and the ways in which they were or were not compromised in your study. You should state your limitations, confident that you made the best possible methodological choices given your set of practice/research circumstances. Remember, the great limitation of the highly prized RCT is that it removes itself from context. The value of PBR is that it is conducted within context.

DISSEMINATION AND PRESENTATION OF FINDINGS

Once you have spent time considering the meaning of and possible explanations for your results, it is time to share them with others. Researchers refer to this process as "research dissemination". As indicated above, one of the major concerns leveled at evaluation and research is that the findings are not used so they do not influence practice and programming (Patton, 2008). While the evidence-based practice movement has placed greater emphasis on social workers accessing research findings to guide practice, there still appears to be a disconnect between research and practice (Epstein, 2009).

Indeed, much of our motivation for engaging practitioners in the research enterprise comes from our prior experience as "outside" evaluators who've had our findings and explanations politely rejected and practice recommendations ignored. Probably for similar reasons, Patton introduced the notion of utilization-focused evaluation in 1978 with the intention of generating evaluation findings that actually get used by decision-makers. Yet, a similar focus has not specifically emerged in relation to social work research. Here, we go one step further than Patton, which is why we think that in PBR practitioners should be fully involved in the interpretation and dissemination phases of any collaborative research effort.

Whether an evaluation researcher or a practitioner-researcher, the way in which you present your findings depends entirely on with whom you are sharing them. The goal is to match your presentation format with your audience. In fact, you will present your findings in quite different ways, so as to maximize the chances that they will be both understood and potentially useful to each particular audience. So first let's consider your potential audience and then we will discuss some ideas about effective presentation style. Here however, it is important to emphasize we are not talking about presenting different sets of findings to please different audiences. Rather we are talking about how to communicate most effectively your findings to your intended audience. There's no point in attempting to "wow" a research-reluctant or unsophisticated audience with fancy statistics.

AUDIENCE

When sharing your study findings your PBR purpose is not to impress but to inform practice and programming. There are a range of different "stakeholders" that might be interested in your results – for example, your clients (or the people you studied), your colleagues, your administrators, colleagues and administrators at other agencies, academics and present or future potential funding sources.

You might access these different audiences via in-person or web-based presentations through a variety of different venues such as within an agency, through a professional organization, or at a conference. Or you might access your audience via a range of different publication options, such as newsletters, short reports (agency website), op-ed (or reader-response) newspaper pieces, policy "white papers", or peer-reviewed academic journal articles.

Understanding that as a practitioner your priorities and time-pressures are different from the ones we have as academics, we still recommend that you share your findings in as many different venues as possible. This allows your PBR study to serve as a catalyst for programming and practice, and your thinking about your study to evolve as dialogue develops. Given the variety of venues and publication types, it makes sense that there is a range of different formats that may be appropriate. In the next section we will discuss how to match your format to your audience and distribution venue.

In conducting workshops and seminars on disseminating results with social workers, one of the things that we put stock in is saying that if you want to be heard, you must also listen. Listen to what your audience is interested in and what they care about – then speak to those things first. In this way you get their attention and find common ground. Once you have done that, then you can share the information that you think is really important about your findings. This is really just another way of saying "know your audience", which is the dissemination equivalent of "be where the client is". Be aware whether your audience is focused on financial concerns or compliance criteria, or charting, or practice, or outcomes. What language and metaphors do they use? Do they want "nuts and bolts", "bottom lines", "process", "cause–effect", or what else? Get a sense of what drives them and then you can find a way to communicate effectively with them.

FORMAT

Effectively communicating your study results is a crucial aspect of the PBR process. Otherwise, why bother? In fact, you will find that working at communicating clearly and effectively to others will make your findings, their limitations and their implications clearer to you.

As we have pointed out throughout this chapter, in PBR the focus of dissemination is on making the results of your study available physically and intellectually so that they can be utilized to inform practice and programming, by an audience of practitioners who may be as close as within your own agency or as far away as the other side of the world (or any other international location). The formats you choose to use will influence the success of that communication. Since it is beyond the scope of this book to give a workshop on verbal presentations, we will focus on print versions of your findings or "visual aids" that may accompany a presentation.

There are three main ways to present your findings, using charts, using tables, or through narrative description. Narrative description may be anything from a short one-page executive summary to a lengthy report with statistical and methodological appendices. Often a combination of charts, tables and narrative can be effective since each person responds differently to information, some responding more to visual cues and others to narrative discussions with case illustrations.

Charts

A chart is a visual representation of information that can serve as a summary of a variable (or a few variables) from your study. Charts have become increasingly easy to generate and can be quite sophisticated and colorful. Some programs are now even able to animate aspects of your charts to show different parts. As the saying goes "a picture tells a thousand words", and so is the case with the right chart. However, the key here is the "right" chart. The wrong picture can be really confusing (see Figure 13.4).

There are some basic rules that we can share about charts, but the rest tends to be subjective. We will start with the rules. Just as some statistical tests are appropriate to use with variables of some levels of measurement and not others, so is the case with charts. For example, in Chapter 12 we discussed why calculating a mean makes sense for an interval level variable, but not for a nominal level variable. The same logic can be applied to bar charts and histograms. While a bar chart (Figure 13.1) looks quite similar to a histogram (Figure 13.3), there is an important distinction. On the bar chart in Figure 13.1 you can see that the categories along the x-axis (the bottom) of the chart are each discrete categories. The order of the categories can be changed without affecting the accuracy of the chart. So, the bar representing Republicans and the one representing Independents could switch places without changing the meaning of the chart. However, the x-axis of the histogram represents the actual scale on which the variable is measured, which is number of years in Figure 13.3. Because the histogram has a continuous scale along the bottom there are blank spaces in the chart where there are no participants representing a particular value, which is not the case for bar charts, which simply omit values that are not represented in the data set. So, as long as you know your level of data, you know whether you want a bar chart or a histogram. Of course, you may want a pie chart and that is a whole other story!

Figures 13.1 and 13.2 display nominal data for political affiliation in two different formats, utilizing a bar chart (Figure 13.1) above and a pie chart (Figure 13.2) below. In many ways personal preference plays a large part in deciding which format you will use. Try different ways and see which one seems to "tell your story" the most clearly. The choice between a bar chart and a pie chart is essentially subjective, unless there are a high number of categories. Figure 13.4 shows that in some computer programs (such as Excel and SPSS) a pie chart can have special features to accentuate different pieces of the pie. This can be especially effective if you are trying to highlight a particular aspect of the data, as is the case with the shockingly small number of social workers who reported receiving adequate supervision in the example.

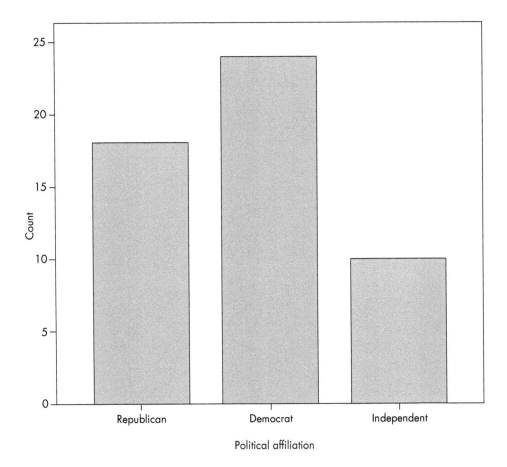

FIGURE 13.1   A bar chart

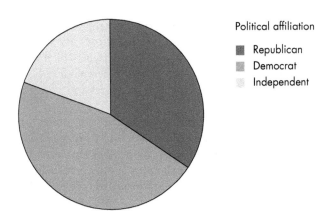

FIGURE 13.2   A pie chart

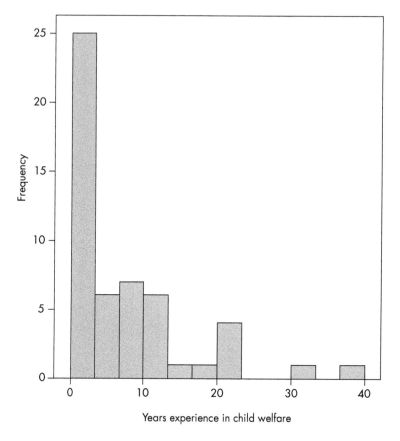

FIGURE 13.3   A histogram

In contrast, Figure 13.5 illustrates why a pie chart might work in some cases but not others. In situations where there are a large number of different scores, representing them in a pie chart tends to be confusing since the pie "slices" are too thin and difficult to read let alone ingest. Figure 13.6 illustrates the way in which a line graph can be especially effective in communicating data across different time points (i.e. change over time). In the case of Figure 13.6, clients' mean depression scores are represented across time at three-month intervals.

Again, the potential to utilize different visual formats reinforces the need to try different types of charts before choosing the one(s) that most clearly represent your data and, ultimately, what you are trying to communicate. Remember that each type of chart is in itself a metaphor that both expresses and in some ways distorts reality. So you need to choose the one that works best for what you are trying to convey and the people to whom you are trying to convey it.

Figures 13.1–13.6 illustrate a few of the different charts available to you for displaying your data. If you spend some time investigating the chart setting in SPSS or taking the tutorial specific to charts you will see that there are numerous other

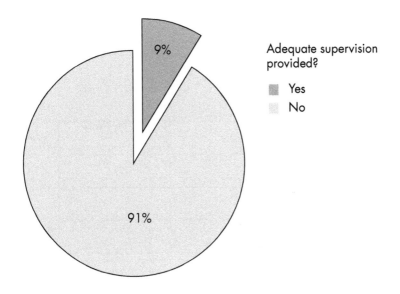

FIGURE 13.4   A pie chart with portion accentuated

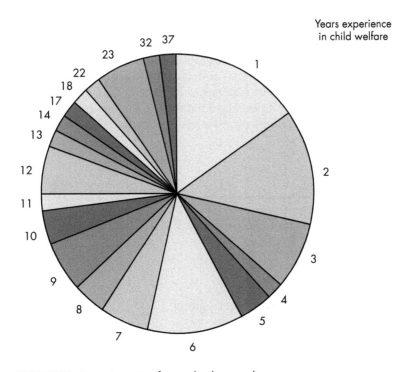

FIGURE 13.5   Learning from a bad example

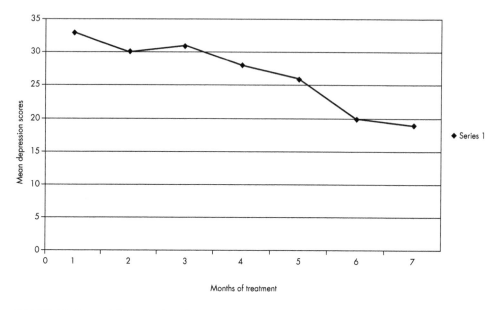

FIGURE 13.6   A line graph – depression over time

alternatives from the very simple to the complex. As you choose which to use heed the advice from Box 13.1, paying special attention to not putting too much information on one chart or graph. The same goes for statistical tables which we will discuss next.

Choosing the right format can really be fun – especially if you are doing it with the assistance of SPSS. Explore the options. The software will never say "no, it's too hard" to you so play with the different possibilities. Have fun with it. Finding creative ways to share your findings with other practitioners and interested parties can be one of the most rewarding aspects of the process.

BOX 13.1   HELPFUL HINTS FOR DISSEMINATION OF RESULTS

Know your purpose
Know your audience
Know your levels of measurement
Don't put too much information on one chart or graph
Titles should be clear and speak for themselves
If it doesn't add to your story or relate to your purpose – leave it out!
Try different things and see which work
Have fun!

Numerical tables

An alternative way to create a graphic representation of data is through the use of numerical tables. The major advantage of tables, is that they can be used to group the results of a series of related questions. Presented instead as a series of many separate pie charts, the reader can get awfully sick of pie. The benefit of tables is that they can accommodate much more information than a chart or a graph without becoming confusing. Table 13.1 provides an example of a table that is being used to display the findings from a research study related to the incorporation of principles from supervision training into practice. By contrast, Table 13.2 illustrates the way in which a large amount of demographic data can be compressed and presented in a way that makes it easy to compare across categories efficiently in a single display.

As with charts, it is important in numerical tables to try presenting different information within the chart in different ways, to see which is the easiest to comprehend and the most aesthetically pleasing presentation. Some rules do apply here, however, as with reporting quantitative data analysis. For example, when giving percentages you should always also note the sample size (N) from which the percentage was generated, and when presenting a mean (*aka* average) score you should also provide the standard deviation so that the reader has a sense of the spread of the scores. (If you don't remember the distinctions between the different measures of central tendency, return briefly to the previous chapter.)

The statistics represented in each cell should be clearly noted at the top of the chart so that the reader knows, for example, whether you are reporting a t-value, an r coefficient or a p-value (ditto for these, see the previous chapter). Also, as with charts it is important in numerical tables to make sure that the title is clear and provides a comprehensive explanation of the content of the table. Finally, as with charts, don't put too much information on one table. The goal is to make the information clear and easy to follow.

TABLE 13.1   Practice areas impacted by supervision training

	Overall rating Mean (SD)	Supported job duties Mean (SD)	Improved knowledge Mean (SD)	Use skills in practice % Yes (n)	Use to train staff % Yes (n)
Learning circles in Year 3 (n = 80)	4.99 (0.11)	4.85 (0.53)	4.86 (0.52)	86 (36)	97 (36)
Train the trainers in Year 3 (n = 24)	5.0 (0.0)	4.79 (0.51)	4.96 (0.20)	70 (10)	90 (10)
All training programs during the 3 years combined (n = 290)	4.9 (0.29)	4.74 (0.44)	4.84 (0.53)	84.9 (167)	85 (167)

TABLE 13.2   Demographic table illustration

	2004 (%, N = 255)	2006 (%, N = 160)
Gender		
Female	82	82
Male	18	18
Race		
African American	20	21
Caucasian	50	46
Latino/Hispanic	18	14
Asian	5	9
Biracial and other	8	5
Age		
20–25	26	11
26–30	31	30
31–35	15	21
36–40	6	6
41+	22	32
Sexual orientation		
Heterosexual	86	82
Lesbian/gay	9	12
Bisexual	4	6
Relationship status		
Married	24	38
Living with s/o	15	13
Divorced	5	3
Single	48	37
Political beliefs		
Liberal	60	54
Conservative	5	7
Moderate	18	16
Radical	12	12
Other	5	7

Narrative

Narratives communicate findings in the form of a story. Obviously qualitative data lend themselves best to a narrative representation. However, writing a summary description of your quantitative findings in words or discussing their practice implications necessarily involves composing a narrative.

Either way, when writing any narrative you need to make a decision whether the style of your sentence structure is going to be short or long, and simple or complex. If the latter is required, it should never be long-winded and flowery. The second author of this book well remembers his advisor's good advice in response to his first draft of his PhD dissertation. "Epstein" he said, "you're not writing a Greek tragedy. So say what you have to say and get the hell out!" We are trying to make the same point a bit more sensitively.

So, you have to make a decision based on what fits your personal writing style, the format of the publication you may be writing for, and your ideas about the preferences of your audience. If possible it is a good idea to get a copy of previous newsletters, reports, or articles that have been published so that they can serve as a guide. While some people think it is important to report research findings in a formal tone, be careful not to create too much formality and distance from your audience, particularly if they are not academics.

Once you have created a first draft of your paper then the process of revising and editing begins. It is very important to create a clean copy of your report because you do not want people to be distracted by mistakes, or to question your study because you made simple errors. "Spell-check" is a good idea but you can't rely entirely on it. Some fairly spectacular goofs have been made as a result of doing so. The computer only knows whether you've spelled a word correctly or not, not whether you've chosen the write word (get it?). Another embarrassment in the academic life history of the second author involved publication of a paper in which the words "anal" and "annals" were interchanged. Both were spelled correctly. (Didn't anything embarrassing ever happen to the first author?)

Even though we both often use the terms revising and editing interchangeably, there is a distinction. Revising refers to the process of adding and deleting new ideas, and changing the structure and order of sentences, while editing refers to checking the spelling, grammar, and matching tenses, etc. Investing time on revisions and edits is an important part of the dissemination process.

A FINAL NOTE ON COLLABORATION

Whether, dear reader, you are a social work research student or a fully-launched practitioner or both, now that you've read our book we think you are ready for us to let you in on an unembarrassing secret from our academic lives. Before even thinking about writing this book together, we did a professional presentation in which we extended a model of academic researcher–practitioner collaboration first developed by McKay and Paikoff (2007). Their "collaborative" model identified various stages of practice-research study development that should by now be quite familiar to you. However, their model of "collaboration" implied that at each stage, the researcher was the key decision-maker and the practitioner was the implementer of those decisions.

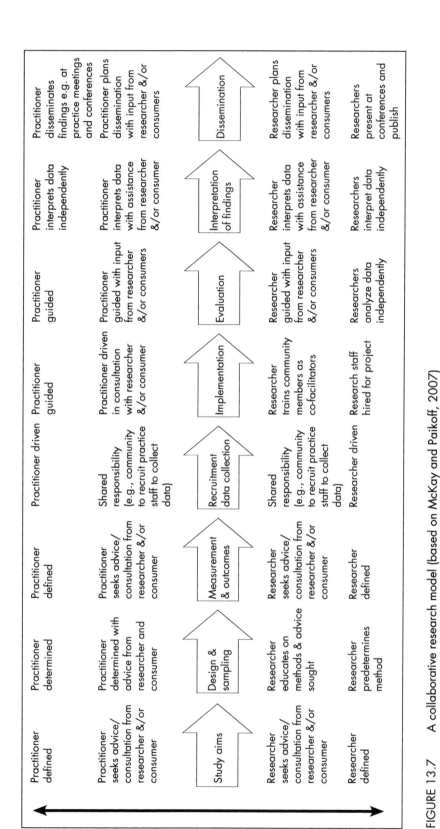

FIGURE 13.7　A collaborative research model (based on McKay and Paikoff, 2007)

Our revision of their model is presented in Figure 13.7. In that figure, we are hoping to convey a model of collaboration in which researcher and practitioner are full partners in decision-making. Our decision to write this book, was fuelled by our desire to empower practitioners to take on this challenge. You can see from the figure, as you have read throughout this book, we firmly believe in the multi-directional nature of collaboration and the centrality of the practitioner in the knowledge generation process. PBR is the vehicle that we hope will take you there.

SUMMARY OF KEY CONCEPTS

In this chapter we have discussed the final but equally important PBR stages of interpretation and dissemination of results. We asserted the value of practitioner wisdom as a key part of the interpretation process, so that the results can be understood within the context of the practice arena from which it was drawn. We also discussed dissemination of results and focusing on matching your presentation method with your audience. We discussed a range of venues where you may present your results, such as within your agency, within professional organizations, and at professional conferences. We also explored different venues for print reports such as newsletters, websites, and journals. We provided examples of three different ways in which results can be presented in print utilizing charts, tables, and narrative or a combination of all three. And we encouraged you to experiment with different formats to see which most effectively display your data. Whatever combination of formats you use we recommend that you try to do as Neuman (2007) suggests by providing a "complete picture of the data without overwhelming the reader" (p.352).

We have concluded with a graphic representation of a model of collaboration in which practitioners and researchers are full partners in every stage of practice–research collaboration. As you set out on your own practice-research journey we wish the very best of luck and encourage you to contact us if you have questions, concerns, would like clarification, or would like to share your really cool PBR study with us!

ADDITIONAL RESOURCES

WEB-BASED RESOURCES

www.googlescholar.com Google Scholar

Quantitative software packages

http://stattrek.com/Tables/Random.aspx website for generating random numbers
http://www.researchinfo.com/docs/calculators/samplesize.cfm website for calculating sample size
http://grants.nih.gov/grants/policy/coc Certificates of Confidentiality
http://www.citiprogram.org Human subjects training course
www.spss.com SPSS

Qualitative software packages

http://www.atlasti.com Atlas.ti
http://www.qsrinternational.com/products_nvivo.aspx NVivo

OTHER RESOURCES

Mertens, D. and Ginsberg, P. (2009) *The Handbook of Social Research Ethics*. Thousand Oaks CA: Sage Publications Inc.
An excellent series of SPSS Manuals is available authored predominantly by Marija Norusis.

REFERENCES

Aisenberg, E. (2008) Evidence-based practice in mental health care to ethnic minority communities: has its practice fallen short of its evidence? *Social Work*, 53 (4): 297–306.

Alexander, L.B. and Solomon, P. (2006) *The Research Process: Behind the scenes*. Toronto: Thomson.

Anastas, J. (1999) *Research Design for Social Work and the Human Services*, 2nd edition. New York: Columbia University Press.

APA (American Psychiatric Association) (2000) *DSM IV – TR Diagnostic and Statistical Manual*, 4th edition (Text Revision). Washington DC: APA.

Beck, A.T., Steer, R.A., Ball, R. and Ranieri, W. (1996) Comparison of Beck Depression Inventories -IA and -II in psychiatric outpatients. *Journal of Personality Assessment*, 67 (3): 588–97.

Beckett, C. and Clegg, S. (2007) Qualitative data from a postal questionnaire: questioning the presumption of value of presence. *International Journal of Social Research Methodology*, 10 (4): 307–17.

Beder, J. (2008) Evaluation research on social work interventions: a study on the impact of social work staffing. *Social Work in Health Care*, 47 (1): 1–13.

Belmont Report (1978) *Ethical Guidelines for the Protection of Human Subjects Research*. Washington, DC: Government Printing Office.

Berk, R.A. (2005) Randomized experiments as the bronze standard. *Journal of Experimental Criminology*, 1 (4): 417–33.

Berlin, S. (1990) Dichotomous and complex thinking. *Social Service Review*, 64 (1): 46–59.

Beutler, L. (2009) Making science matter in clinical practice: redefining psychotherapy. *Clinical Psychology: Science and Practice*, 16 (4): 301–17.

Bloom, M., Fischer, J. and Orme, J. (1995) *Evaluating Practice: Guidelines for the accountable professional*, 2nd edition. Boston: Allyn & Bacon.

Blumenfield, S. and Epstein, I. (2001) Introduction: promoting and maintaining a reflective professional staff in a hospital-based social work department. *Social Work in Health Care*, 33 (3/4): 1–14.

Boehmer, U. (2002) Twenty years of public health research: Inclusion of lesbian, gay, bisexual and transgender populations. *American Journal of Public Health*, 92 (7): 1125–30.

Brekke, J., Ell, K. and Palinkas, L. (2007) Translational science at the National Institute of Mental Health: can social work take its rightful place? *Research on Social Work Practice*, 17 (1): 123–33.

Briar, S. (1979) Incorporating research into education for clinical practice in social work: toward a clinical science in social work. In A. Rubin and A. Rosenblatt (eds) *Sourcebook on Research Utilization*. New York: Council on Social Work Education.

Campbell, D. and Stanley, J. (1963) *Experimental and Quasi-Experimental Designs for Research*. Chicago: Rand McNally.

Ceci, S., Peters, D. and Plotkin, J. (1985) Human subjects review, personal values, and the regulation of social science research. *American Psychologist*, 40 (9): 994–1002.

Chan, W.C.H., Epstein, I., Reese, D. and Chan, C.L.W. (2009) Family predictors of psychosocial outcomes among Hong Kong Chinese cancer patients in palliative care: living and dying with the support paradox. *Social Work in Health Care*, 48 (5): 519–32.

Cherin, D. and Meezan, W. (1998) Evaluation as a means of organizational learning. *Administration in Social Work*, 22 (2): 1–21.

Cordero, A. (2000) When reunification works: a family strengths perspective. Unpublished doctoral dissertation: Graduate Faculty in Social Welfare. The City University of New York.

Cordero, A. and Epstein, I. (2005) Refining the practice of reunification: "mining" successful foster care case records of substance abusing families. In G.P. Mallon and P.M. Hess (eds) *Child Welfare for the Twenty-First Century: A handbook of practices, policies and programs.* New York: Columbia University Press.

Craft, J. (1990) *Statistics and Data Analysis for Social Workers*, 2nd edition. Itasca, IL: F.E. Peacock Publishers.

Creswell, J. (2009) *Research Design: Qualitative, quantitative, and mixed methods approaches*, 3rd edition. Thousand Oaks, CA: Sage Publications Inc.

CSWE (2008) *Educational Policy and Accreditation Standards*. Washington DC: Council on Social Work Education.

De Grunchy, J. and Lewin, S. (2001) Ethics that exclude: the role of ethics committees in lesbian and gay health research in South Africa. *American Journal of Public Health*, 91 (6): 865–8.

Denzin, N. and Lincoln, Y. (eds) (2008) *The Landscape of Qualitative Research*, 3rd edition. Thousand Oaks CA: Sage Publications Inc.

Dobrof, J., Dolinko, A., Lichtiger, E., Uribarri, J. and Epstein, I. (2001) Dialysis patient characteristics and outcomes: the complexity of social work practice with end stage renal disease. *Social Work in Health Care*, 33 (3/4): 105–28.

Dobrof, J., Ebenstein, H., Dodd, S.J. and Epstein, I. (2006) Caregivers and professionals partnership: assessing a hospital support program for family caregivers. *Journal of Palliative Medicine*, 9 (1): 196–205.

Dodd, S. (2009) LGBTQ: Protecting vulnerable subjects in all studies. In D. Mertons and P. Ginsberg (eds) *Handbook of Social Science Research Ethics*. Thousand Oaks, CA: Sage Publications.

Dodd, S.J. and Epstein, I. (2006) Meeting the challenge of research-practice integration: conducting practice-based research in and with diverse communities. Paper presented at the 10th Annual Conference of the Society for Social Work and Research, San Antonio, Texas.

Dodd, S.J. and Meezan, W. (2009) Matching AIDS service organizations' philosophy of service provision with a compatible style of program evaluation. In W. Meezan and J. Martin (eds) *Handbook of Research with Lesbian, Gay, Bisexual, and Transgender Populations.* New York: Harrington Park Press.

Dolgoff, R. and Skolnick, L. (1992) Ethical decision making, the NASW Code of Ethics and groupwork practice: beginning explorations. *Social Work with Groups*, 15 (4): 99–112.

Encarta World English Computer Based Dictionary.

Epstein, I. (1987) Pedagogy of the perturbed: teaching research to the reluctants. *Journal of Teaching in Social Work*, 1: 71–89.

Epstein, I. (1995) Promoting reflective social work practice: research strategies and consulting principles. In P. Hess and E. Mullens (eds) *Practitioner-Researcher Partnerships: Building knowledge from, in and for practice.* Washington DC: NASW Press.

Epstein, I. (1996) In quest of a research-based model for clinical practice: or, why can't a social worker be more like a researcher? *Social Work Research*, 20: 97–100.

Epstein, I. (2001) Using available clinical information in practice-based research: mining for silver while dreaming of gold. In I. Epstein and S. Blumenfield (eds) *Clinical Data-Mining in Practice-Based Research: Social work in hospital settings.* Binghamton NY: Haworth Press.

Epstein, I. (2005) Following in the footnotes of giants: citation analysis and its discontents. *Social Work in Healthcare*, 41 (3/4): 93–101.

Epstein, I. (2007) From evaluation methodologist to clinical data-miner: finding treasure through practice-based research. In H. Rehr and G. Rosenberg (eds) *The Social Work–Medicine Relationship: 100 years at Mount Sinai*. Binghamton, NY: Haworth Press.

Epstein, I. (2009) Promoting harmony where there is commonly conflict: evidence-informed practice as an integrative strategy. *Social Work in Health Care*, 48 (3): 216–31.

Epstein, I. (2010) *Clinical Data-Mining: Integrating practice and research*. New York: Oxford University Press.

Epstein, I. (2011) "Commentary". Reconciling evidence-based practice, evidence-informed practice and practice-based research: the role of clinical data-mining. *Social Work*.

Epstein, I. and Blumenfield, S. (eds) (2001) *Clinical Data-Mining in Practice-Based Research: Social work in hospital settings*. New York: Routledge.

Epstein, I. and Conrad, K. (1978) The empirical limits of social work professionalization. In R. Sarri and Y. Hasenfeld (eds) *The Management of Human Services*. New York: Columbia University Press.

Epstein, I. and Hench, C. (1979) Behavior modification in the classroom: education or social control? *Journal of Sociology and Social Welfare*, 6 (5): 223–9.

Epstein, I., Lalayants, M., Auslander, G., Chan, W., Fouche, F., Giles, R., Joubert, L., Rosenne, H. and Vertigan, A. (2011) Globalize the methodology, localize the findings: clinical data-mining in international settings. Unpublished manuscript submitted to *The International Journal of Social Work*.

Epstein, I. and Tripodi, T. (1978) *Research Techniques for Program Planning, Monitoring and Evaluation*. New York: Columbia University Press.

Fischer, J. and Corcoran, K. (2007) *Measures for Clinical Practice: A sourcebook*, 4th edition. New York: Oxford University Press.

Fisher, C., Reece, M., Dodge, B., Wright, E., Sherwood-Laughlin, C. and Baldwin, K. (2010) Expanding our reach: the potential for youth development professionals in community-based organizations to provide sexuality information. *American Journal of Sexuality Education*, 5 (1): 36–53.

Galtung, J. (1967) *Theory and Methods of Social Research*. New York: Columbia University Press.

Gambrill, E. (1995) Less marketing more scholarship. *Social Work Research*, 19 (1): 38–47.

Gambrill, E. (2006) Evidence-based practice and policy: choices ahead. *Research on Social Work Practice*, 16 (3): 338–57.

Gambrill, E. (2010) Evidence-informed practice: Antidote to propaganda in the helping professions? *Research on Social Work Practice*, 20: 302–20.

Gambrill, E. and Gibbs, L.E. (2009) *Critical Thinking for Helping Professionals: A skills based workbook*, 3rd edition. New York: Oxford University Press.

Germain, C.B. (1991) *Human Behavior in the Social Environment: An ecological view*. New York: Columbia University Press.

Gibbs, L. and Gambrill, E. (2002) Evidence-based practice: counter arguments and objections. *Research on Social Work Practice*, 12: 452–76.

Glaser, B. and Strauss, A. (1967) *The Discovery of Grounded Theory: Strategies for qualitative research*. Chicago: Aldine Publishing Company.

Goffman, E. (1961) *Asylums: Essays on the social situation of mental patients*. New York: Doubleday & Co.

Goodman, H. (2001) In-depth interviews. In B.A.Thyer (ed) *The Handbook of Social Work Research Methods*. Thousand Oaks, CA: Sage Publications Inc.

Grasso, A.J. and Epstein, I. (1992) (eds) *Research Utilization in the Social Services: Innovations for practice and administration*. Binghamton NY: Haworth Press.

Guba, E. (1990) *The Paradigm Dialog*. Thousand Oaks CA: Sage Publications Inc.

Guba, E. and Lincoln, Y. (1989) *Fourth Generation Evaluation*. Thousand Oaks CA: Sage Publications Inc.

Guba, E. and Lincoln, Y. (1994) Competing paradigms in qualitative research. In N. Denzin and Y. Lincoln (eds) *The Landscape of Qualitative Research*. Thousand Oaks CA: Sage Publications Inc.

Guba, E. and Lincoln, Y. (2008) Paradigmatic controversies, contradictions and emerging confluences. In N. Denzin and Y. Lincoln (eds) *The Landscape of Qualitative Research* (3rd edition). Thousand Oaks CA: Sage Publications Inc.

Halmos, P. (1970) *The Personal Service Society*. London: Constable.

Hamilton, M. (1980) Rating depressive patients. *Journal of Clinical Psychiatry*, 41: 21–4.

Hanssen, D. and Epstein, I. (2007) Learning what works: demonstrating practice effectiveness with children and families through retrospective investigation. *Family Preservation*, 10: 24–41.

Harder, J. (2010) Overcoming MSW students' reluctance to engage in research. *Journal of Teaching in Social Work*, 30 (2): 195–209.

Heineman, M. (1981) The obsolete scientific imperative in social work research. *Social Service Review*, 55: 391.

Heineman Pieper, M. (1985) The future of social work research. *Social Work Research and Abstracts*, 21: 3–11.

Heineman Pieper, M. (1986) Some common misunderstandings of the heuristic approach. *Social Work Research and Abstracts*, 22 (2): 22

Hill-Collins, P. (1990) *Black Feminist Thought*. Boston: Unwin Hyman.

Howe, K. (2004) A critique of experimentalism. *Qualitative Inquiry*, 10: 42–61.

Hudson, W. (1982) Scientific imperatives in social work research practice. *Social Service Review*, 56 (2): 246–57.

Humphreys, L. (1970) *Tearoom Trade: Impersonal sex in public places*. New York: Aldine.

Hutchison, E.D. (2008) *Dimensions of Human Behavior: Person and environment*, 3rd edition. Thousand Oaks CA: Sage Publications Inc.

Hutson, C. and Lichtiger, E. (2001) Mining clinical information in the utilization of social services: practitioners inform themselves. *Social Work in Health Care*, 33 (3/4): 153–62.

Imre, R. (1985) Tacit knowledge in social work research and practice. *Smith College Studies in Social Work*, 55 (2): 13–49.

Ivanoff, A., Blythe, B. and Briar, S. (1997) What's the story, Morning Glory? *Social Work Research*, 21 (3): 194–6.

Jones, J. (1993) *Bad Blood: The Tuskegee Syphilis Experiment*. New York: Free Press.

Jones, S., Statham, H. and Solomou, W. (2006) When expectant mothers know their baby has a fetal abnormality: exploring a crisis of motherhood through qualitative data mining. *Journal of Social Work Research and Evaluation*, 6 (2): 195–206.

Joubert, L. and Epstein, I. (eds) (2005) Special Issue. Multi-disciplinary data-mining in allied health practice: another perspective on Australian research and evaluation. *Journal of Social Work Research and Evaluation*, 6 (2): 139–41.

Keyser, D. and Sweetland, R. (2004) *Test Critiques*. Austin TX: Pro-Ed.

Kirk, S.A. and Reid, W. (2002) *Science and Social Work*. New York: Columbia University Press.

Kitchener, K. and Kitchener, R. (2009) Social science research ethics: historical and philosophical issues. In D. Mertons and P. Ginsberg (eds) *Handbook of Social Science Research Ethics*. Thousand Oaks CA: Sage Publications Inc.

Littell, J., Corcoran, J. and Pillai, V. (2008) *Systematic Reviews and Meta-Analysis*. New York: Oxford University Press.

Lo, H.M., Epstein, I., Ng, S.M., Chan, C.L., Ho, C.S. (in press) When cognitive behavioral group therapy works and when it doesn't: clinical data mining on CBGT outcomes for depression and anxiety among Hong Kong Chinese. *Social Work in Mental Health*.

Loutzenheiser, L. (2007) Working alterity: the impossibility of ethical research with youth. *Educational Studies*, 41 (2): 109–27.

Matthews, J. and Cramer, E. (2008) Using technology to enhance qualitative research with hidden populations. *The Qualitative Report*, 13 (2): 301–15.

McCracken, S. and Marsh, J.C. (2008) Practitioner expertise in evidence-based practice decision-making. *Research on Social Work Practice*, 18 (4): 301–10.

McCubbin, H. (1998) *Stress, Coping and Health in Families: Sense of coherence and resiliency.* Thousand Oaks CA: Sage Publications Inc.

McKay, M. and Paikoff, R. (eds) (2007) *Community Collaborative Partnerships: The Foundation for HIV Prevention Research Efforts.* New York: Taylor & Francis.

McNeece, A. and Thyer, B. (2004) Evidence-based practice and social work. *Journal of Evidence-Based Social Work*, 1: 7–25.

McNeill, T. (2006) Evidence-based practice in an age of relativism. *Social Work*, 51 (2): 147–56.

Milgram, S. (1974) *Obedience to Authority: An experimental view.* New York: Harper Collins.

Mirabito, D. (2000) Keeping the door open or keeping the door shut? How and why adolescents terminate from mental health treatment. Unpublished doctoral dissertation: Graduate faculty in Social Welfare. The City University of New York.

Monette, D., Sullivan, T. and DeJong, C. (1994) *Applied Social Research: Tools for the human services*, 3rd edition. Fort Worth: Harcourt Brace College Publishers.

Mullen, E.J. (2004) Facilitating practitioner use of evidence-based practice. In A.E. Roberts and K.R. Yeager (eds) *Evidence-Based Practice Manual: Research and outcome measures in health and human services.* New York: Oxford University Press.

Myers, L. and Thyer, B. (1997) Should social work clients have the right to effective treatment? *Social Work*, 42 (3): 288–98.

NASW (2008) *Code of Ethics of the National Association of Social Workers* (revised) Washington, DC: NASW.

Nevo, I. and Slonim-Nevo V. (2011) The myth of evidence-based practice: towards evidence-informed practice. *British Journal of Social Work*, 41 (1): 1–22.

Neuman, W. (2007) *The Basics of Social Research: Qualitative and quantitative approaches.* Boston MA: Pearson Education, Inc.

Padgett, D. (1998) *Qualitative Methods in Social Work Research: Challenges and rewards.* Thousand Oaks CA: Sage Publications Inc.

Patton, M. (2008) *Utilization Focused Evaluation*, 4th edition. Thousand Oaks CA: Sage Publications Inc.

Peake, K., Epstein, I. and Medeiros, D. (eds) (2005) *Clinical and Research Uses of an Adolescent Intake Questionnaire: What kids need to talk about.* Binghamton NY: Haworth Press.

Peile, C. (1988) Research paradigms in social work: From stalemate to creative synthesis. *Social Service Review*, 6 (2): 1–19.

Pignotti, M. and Thyer, B. (2009) Use of novel unsupported and empirically supported therapies by Licensed Clinical Social Workers: an exploratory study. *Social Work Research*, 33 (1): 5–17.

Plath, D.A. and Gibbons, J.L. (2010) Discoveries on a data-mining expedition: single session social work in hospitals. *Social Work in Health Care*, 49: 703–17.

Polsky, H.W. (1977) *Cottage Six: Social system of delinquent boys in residential treatment.* New York: Krieger.

Rajudaran, S. (2011) Filipino women domestics on an international economic mission: a multi-method, data-mining study. Unpublished PhD Dissertation: Graduate Faculty in Social Welfare, City University of New York.

Random House (1980) *The Random House College Dictionary Revised Edition.* New York: Random House Inc.

Reeser, L. and Epstein, I. (1990) *Professionalization and Activism in Social Work: The 60s, the 80s and the future.* New York: Columbia University Press.

Ripple, L. (1960) Problem identification and formulation. In N. Polansky (ed) *Social Work Research.* Chicago IL: University of Chicago Press.

Roberts, A.E. and Yeager, K. R. (2004) Systematic reviews of evidence-based studies and prac-tice-based research: how to search for, develop, and use them. In A.E. Roberts and K.R. Yeager (eds) *Evidence-Based Practice Manual: Research and outcome measures in health and human services*. New York: Oxford University Press.

Royse, D., Staton-Tindall, M., Badger, K. and Webster, M. (2009) *Needs Assessment*. New York: Oxford University Press.

Rubin, A. (2008) *Practitioner's Guide to Using Research for Evidence-Based Practice*. Hoboken NJ: John Wiley & Sons.

Rubin, A. and Babbie, E. (1993) *Research Methods for Social Work*, 2nd edition. Pacific Grove CA: Brooks/Cole Publishing Co.

Sacks, J. (1985) Specific strategies of problem formulation: a gap in our methods? *Smith College Studies in Social Work*, 55 (3): 214–24.

Saini, M. and Shlonsky, A. (in press) *Systematic Syntheses of Qualitative Research*. New York: Oxford University Press.

Sainz, A. and Epstein, I. (2001) Creating experimental analogs with available clinical informa-tion: credible alternatives to "gold standard" experiments? *Social Work in Health Care*, 33 (3/4): 163–84.

Saleeby, D. (ed) (2008) *The Strengths Perspective in Social Work Practice,* 5th edition. Boston: Allyn & Bacon.

Sales, E., Lichtenwalter, S. and Fevola, A. (2006) Secondary analysis in social work research education: past, present, and future promise. *Journal of Social Work Education*, 42 (3): 543–58.

Schmidt, A. (2010) Prevalence, Predictors and Negative Outcomes Associated with Discordant Sexual Identity, Sexual Attraction and Sexual Behavior. Unpublished doctoral dissertation: Graduate faculty in Social Welfare. The City University of New York.

Schon, D. (1983) *The Reflective Practitioner: How professionals think in action*. New York: Basic Books.

Scriven, M. (1995) The logic of evaluation and evaluation practice. In D.M. Fournier (ed) *Reasoning in Evaluation: Inferential links and leaps*. San Francisco: Jossey-Bass.

Sieber, J. (2004) Empirical research on research ethics. *Ethics and Behavior*, 14 (4): 397–412.

Stoesz, D. (2010) Second rate research for second class citizens. *Research on Social Work Practice*, 20: 329–32.

Tripodi, T., and Lalayants, M. (2008) Research overview. In T. Mizrahi and L.E. Davis (eds) *Encyclopedia of Social Work*, 20th edition. New York: Oxford University Press.

Tutty, L., Rothery, M. and Grinnell, R. (1996) *Qualitative Research for Social Workers*. Boston: Allyn & Bacon.

United States Census Bureau (2000) www.census.gov/main/www/cen2000.html

Vonk, E., Tripodi, T. and Epstein, I. (2006) *Research Techniques for Clinical Social Workers*, 2nd edition. New York: Columbia University Press.

Weinbach, R. and Grinnell, R. (2001) *Statistics for Social Workers*, 5th edition. Boston: Pearson, Allyn & Bacon.

Weinbach, R. and Grinnell, R. (2010) *Statistics for Social Workers*, 8th edition. Boston: Pearson, Allyn & Bacon.

Wilson, W. and Rosenthal, B. (1993) Anxiety and performance in an MSW research and statis-tics course. *Journal of Teaching in Social Work*, 6 (2): 75–85.

Yegedis, B. and Weinbach, R. (2002) *Research Methods for Social Workers*, 4th edition. Boston: Allyn & Bacon.

Yegedis, B. and Weinbach, R. (2008) *Research Methods for Social Workers*, 6th edition. Boston: Allyn & Bacon.

Yesavage, J.A., Brink, T.L., Rose, T.L., Lum, O., Huang, V., Adey, M.B. and Leirer, V.O. (1983) Development and validation of a geriatric depression screening scale: a preliminary report. *Journal of Psychiatric Research*, 17: 37–49.

Zilberfein, F., Hutson, C., Snyder, S. and Epstein, I. (2001) Social work practice with pre- and post-liver transplant patients: a retrospective self-study. *Social Work in Health Care*, 33, (3/4): 91–104.

Zung, W.W.K. (1965) A self-rating depression scale. *Archives of General Psychiatry,* 12: 63–70.

INDEX

Pages containing relevant figures and tables are indicated by *italic* type; material within boxes is indicated by **bold** type.